Thai Yoga Massage

Thai Yoga Massage

A DYNAMIC THERAPY FOR PHYSICAL WELL-BEING AND SPIRITUAL ENERGY

Kam Thye Chow

Healing Arts Press
Rochester, Vermont

To Anika and our children, Keanu and Dana,
with much love,
and
To Thai Yoga Massage,
with gratitude.

❖

Healing Arts Press
One Park Street
Rochester, Vermont 05767
www.InnerTraditions.com

Healing Arts Press is a division of Inner Traditions International

Note to the reader: This book is intended as an informational guide.
The remedies, approaches, and techniques described herein are meant to supplement, and not to be a substitute for, professional medical care or treatment. They should not be used to treat a serious ailment without prior consultation with a qualified health care professional.

THE LIBRARY OF CONGRESS HAS CATALOGED THE HARDCOVER EDITION AS FOLLOWS:
Chow, Kam Thye.
Thai yoga massage : a dynamic therapy for physical well-being and spiritual energy / Kam Thye Chow.
p. cm.
Includes bibliographical references.
ISBN 0-89281-937-5
1. Massage therapy. 2. Yoga, Hatha. 3. Medicine, Thai. I. Title.
RM721 .C48 2002
615.8'22—dc21
2001051947

ISBN of paperback with DVD edition: ISBN 0-89281-146-3

Printed and bound in Canada

10   9   8   7   6   5   4   3   2   1

Illustrations by Kam Thye Chow
Photographs by Serge Caron

Text design and layout by Virginia Scott Bowman
This book was typeset in Sabon with Delphin and Civet as the display typefaces

Contents

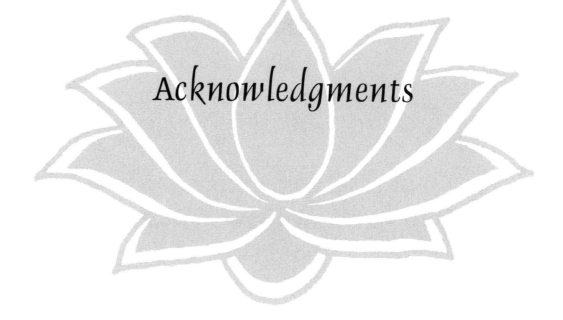

Acknowledgments

I would like to begin by honoring all my teachers who have guided me in my practice and taught me the spiritual notion of *metta* (love and kindness). I am deeply grateful and fortunate to have met such great individuals who have shared their art and knowledge so generously. I particularly want to acknowledge my teacher and friend Asokananda, who provided me with a foundation in Thai Yoga Massage. His landmark research in the sen energy lines has been a great contribution to the field of Thai massage and to this book.

A special thank you to Emily Moody who appeared as an angel and a sister on the path of dharma at the right time. Her dedication and assistance with writing and editing helped me put my thoughts into words. Without her this book would not have been possible.

To my senior student, Pierre Boudreau, who, despite his initial reluctance to learn this art, today is a well-established and reputed teacher and practitioner. To Chris Holmes, whose help in the practical aspect of part 2 was invaluable. His skill as a communicator and teacher of Thai Yoga Massage has enhanced the instructional side of this book considerably. To Lissa Guilbault for her constant support in building the Lotus Palm School. To Tom Casey, whose understanding of dance and movement helped with the overall flow of the book.

Thank you to Serge Caron, my photographer, for his kind and easygoing nature. To

Catherine Waller for her assistance in the charting of the sen energy lines. To Dr. Geraldine Jacquemin, M.D., for her generous medical advice. Thank you to my editor at Healing Arts Press, Susan Davidson, for all her hard work and ability to get this book finished.

My deepest thanks to the love of my life, my wife, Anika Lefebvre, M.D., for her advice and overview on all the medical aspects of the book and for being the model in the photographs. Her constant support and understanding is nothing but pure love. I could not have made this book without her patience, not to mention her trust in allowing me to swing her around in all those Thai yoga postures!

I would like to close by thanking my Indian dance teacher, Prakash, for sharing his ancient story of the cake. Knowledge, he says, is like a piece a cake cut into four quarters. The first piece represents learning from your teacher, the second listening and remembering his or her advice, the third putting the art into practice, and the final piece signifies teaching the art that you have learned. After teaching for a number of years, another cake has developed for me. I have found that my so-called students are now my teachers. They help me to learn, listen, practice, and evolve. So a warm thank-you to all of my students who over the years have helped me to grow as a teacher and develop the Lotus Palm tradition of Thai Yoga Massage.

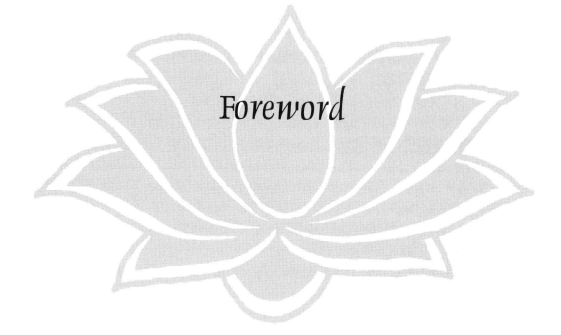

Foreword

I was in Canada directing seminars when a good friend said to me, "You really must meet my friend Kam Thye. He is an extraordinary man with a gift." We arranged a meeting and I received my first Thai Yoga Massage session. I was treated to a blend of pressure-point work, breath awareness, and having my lanky 6'5" frame effortlessly flipped around like a pile of sticks. At the end of the experience I was deeply relaxed and felt keenly attuned to the new flow of energy through my body.

In addition to that masterful session I also received a deeply healing presence embodied by this compact and self-contained man. I asked Kam Thye what he felt was the most important aspect of his work. He smiled broadly and held up his open hands. "It's all *metta*," he replied, referring to the Buddhist practice of loving kindness.

What makes a healer a great healer? Many practitioners have studied technique—they understand physiology and body mechanics, yet fall short of connecting to their clients on a deeper level. Transcendent to all techniques must be purity of heart and a clear intention to serve. That quality is what I have encountered in my years of friendship with Kam Thye Chow.

The mystical blend inherent in Thai Yoga Massage, with its Ayurvedic roots, organic flow of movement, and martial arts–like transitions, reflects Kam Thye Chow's cultural influences. Born in Malaysia into a Chinese family of healers, Kam Thye was immersed from an early age in the world of Chinese martial arts and Buddhist philosophy. He was also profoundly touched by the Indian practices of yoga and Ayurveda.

How does the practice of Thai Yoga Massage today differ from two thousand years ago? One of the compelling aspects of Thai Yoga Massage is how it evolves over time, shaped by the deepening relationship between practitioner and receiver. And yet there is a timelessness to Thai Yoga Massage as well, particularly when it is grounded in the practice of metta. The beauty of Kam Thye's presence is his foundation in the authenticity of this ancient and core practice. I imagine that a great session today differs little from a great session thousands of years ago, assuming the practitioner opens fully to the healing flow of energy and selflessly offers his awareness and presence to the receiver in a constant state of prayer. Love transcends time, and in that space, healing is infinite in its reach.

Over the years Kam Thye and I have shared a yearning toward spirit, and each of us, in his own way, has practiced the life of the monk and wanderer. Now with family, Kam Thye is able to cultivate a spiritual practice while living the life of a householder. At Kripalu Center for Yoga and Health, the largest yoga and health center in North America, we are constantly looking for authentic doorways through which to offer our guests an experience of properly aligning body, mind, and spirit. We are honored to have Kam Thye as a faculty member at Kripalu and have received an overwhelmingly positive response to his teachings. The publication of his book is an important and timely contribution to the field of bodywork and healing.

Buddhism studies how we move from the infinite to the finite; that journey is described as moving from one thing, to two things, to ten thousand things. Our busy and active world is filled with the "ten thousand things" that are constantly calling for our attention. Thai Yoga Massage practitioners focus on an infinite set of variables at one time, performing gentle, dynamic movements with the receiver while attending to her breath rhythm, energy lines, pressure points, and Ayurvedic doshas. To sustain these multiple levels of attention can overwhelm the mind. In my perspective, Kam Thye's gifts as an educator and guide are not only his skill in navigating through the never-ending depth of this bodywork art—the ancient and contemporary practice of Thai Yoga Massage—but how, in the purity of his intention, he brings the practice back from ten thousand things, to two, to one: the practice of metta, the return home to the timelessness of love.

Sudhir Jonathan Foust
President, Kripalu Center for Yoga and Health

PART ONE

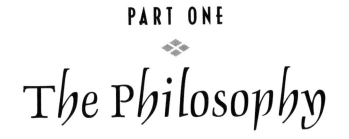

The Philosophy

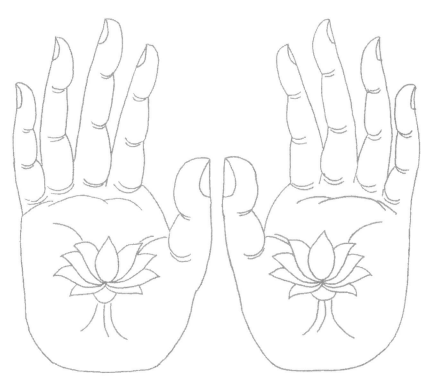

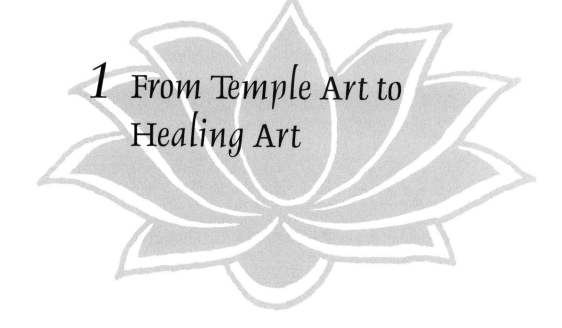

1 From Temple Art to Healing Art

I am from Malaysia, a peninsular nation between China and India. Historically, Malaysia was the meeting place for the great cultures of these two countries. Many merchants, artisans, and laborers who came to the Far East settled in Malaysia; they were accompanied by healers, yogis, martial artists, and herbalists who brought their spiritual beliefs with them.

My family is of Chinese origin. I began studying the traditional Taoist arts of tai chi chuan, chi kung, massage, and herbal healing at the age of thirteen. Growing up in Malaysia, I had Hindu friends from India whose practices of Ayurveda, yoga, massage, and mantra meditation were thoroughly integrated into their lifestyles. I consider myself fortunate to have been brought up in this environment.

I feel even more blessed to have found the art of Thai Yoga Massage, which is a synthesis of yoga, Ayurveda, and meditation. For this I am indebted to my teacher and good friend, Asokananda, with whom I studied in Chang Mai, Thailand, for six years. He generously shared this precious art with me and introduced me to the philosophy of *metta*, loving compassion. Together we have taught Thai Yoga Massage around the world.

Thai Yoga Massage is performed on the floor in loose and comfortable clothing. In receiving Thai Yoga Massage one is also receiving the benefits of the practice of yoga. This technique has been described as assisted Hatha yoga. A Thai Yoga Massage also incorporates martial arts moves, rhythmic motion, palming and thumbing along energy lines, gentle stretching, and breathwork, creating a slow, flowing "dance" around and with the recipient's body.

In addition to stretching and tonifying the muscles, Thai Yoga Massage improves circulation, relieves muscular tension and spasm, helps expedite metabolism, boosts the immune system, and balances the body energetically, inducing a calm mental state. This practice provides the recipient with both a physical and an energetic massage.

—ɯ—

The origins of traditional Thai massage can be traced back 2,500 years to India and the spread of Buddhism. The founding father of Thai massage, Jivaka Kumarbhaccha, was a celebrated yogi and a doctor in the ancient Indian healing tradition of Ayurveda. His unusual skill as a physician and surgeon was so well known that he

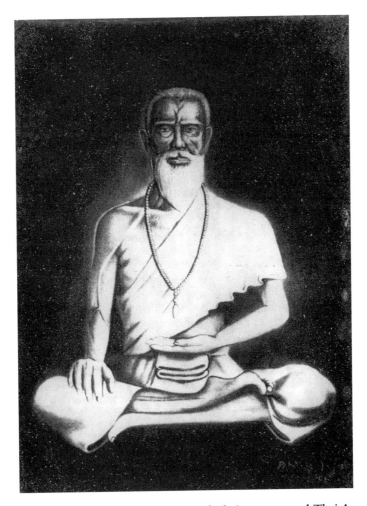

Jivaka Kumarbhaccha, the founding father of Thai massage and Thai Ayurveda

was called upon to treat kings and princes, including the Magadha King Bimbisara. But of all the people Jivaka attended to, the most distinguished was the Buddha. Today, Jivaka is not only venerated as the founder of traditional Thai massage; he is also honored as the source of Ayurvedic practices within Thailand.

Traditional Thai massage developed over centuries within the environment of the Buddhist temples. The Thai temple, or *wat,* also operates as a center for the health care of the common people. The most famous institution for traditional Thai massage is the Wat Pho in Bangkok, still today the leading center of research and practice for the art of Thai massage. In addition to being the main center for the practice of Buddhism in Thailand, Wat Pho temple houses various stone-carved figurines eloquently holding Thai massage postures. The inside walls of the temple bear epigraphs depicting the *sen,* the body's energy line network. Installed by King Rama III in 1832, these famous sculptures and illustrations give visual form to the theoretical foundations of traditional Thai massage healing work.

While traditional Thai massage is a culturally integrated tradition in Thailand, it is difficult to talk about a standard form of Thai massage—various masters have cultivated their own distinct methods of practice. There are, however, two general styles within Thailand that can be traced to the teachings of two main schools: the northern school and the southern school.

Setting the standard for the northern school is the Old Medical Hospital in Chang Mai. At the Old Medical Hospital the day begins with a chant in praise of Jivaka, the founder of Thai massage, to inspire the day's work. In the south, the main teaching center is Wat Pho in Bangkok. The main difference between these two styles is how each technique works with energy lines in the body. The northern style could be said to be a *yang* form, since it is slightly more active in its approach. It emphasizes the techniques of palming and thumbing, the latter being a method that involves the practitioner focusing his bodyweight through his arms and gradually pouring that weight into the recipient to tonify the recipient's energy lines. The southern school, with a slightly more relaxed approach, is more *yin* in nature. It emphasizes the technique of plucking, in which the practitioner uses his fingers to strum or stimulate the nerves running along the energy lines.

As travel between these two regions has increased, the northern and southern styles are becoming increasingly integrated.

This dynamic form of therapeutic massage originated in India and became an integrated aspect of the temple environment within Thailand when Buddhism spread to Southeast Asia. Over the past ten years a growing number of westerners have traveled to Thailand to study massage and have returned to the West to open schools and training centers. As a result, a fusion of many new styles is now being practiced around the world.

After growing up in Malaysia inside the practice of the healing arts and living in Thailand for six years with my Thai massage teacher, Asokananda, I am now settled in Montreal—not a place I thought I would end up!—and am teaching a form of Thai Yoga Massage that I call Lotus Palm Thai Yoga Bodywork. This massage method has recently been recognized by the Féderation quebécoise des massothépeutes (FQM, the Quebec massage federation) and the College of Massage Therapists of Ontario (CMTO). With a foundation in traditional Thai massage concepts, the Lotus Palm method incorporates Ayurvedic principles, the Buddhist attention to centeredness, the alignment and dynamic stretching of Hatha yoga, and manipulation of the sen, the Thai energy line system. Lotus Palm focuses on creating a flowing dance that is characteristic of tai chi, benefiting both the practitioner and receiver.

When explaining this method of Thai Yoga Massage I like to use the image of the tango. Linked together in a graceful dance, the principal dancer (the practitioner) and the follower (the recipient) perform a series of yoga positions. The practitioner uses her hands, feet, arms, and legs to gently guide the recipient into various yoga postures while remaining focused and centered. The more skillful and fluid the practitioner, the more the recipient is able to relax and trust her as the principal dancer. As the dance becomes more beautiful and harmonious, it also becomes more healing and beneficial to the receiver.

Lotus Palm Thai Yoga Bodywork emphasizes centering, transition, balance, safety, and using the least amount of effort to achieve maximum results. There is a strong emphasis on safety and on rhythmic, flowing transitions from one posture to the next. The lotus is a symbol of loving-kindness and compassion, while "palming" is a technique that we use in Thai Yoga Massage. Lotus Palm means "the compassionate touch." That is the spirit of this work.

As has been the case with other Eastern practices introduced to the West, in adapting this art to a new culture changes have been inevitable. The Lotus Palm method teaches a form of Thai massage specifically designed for westerners. People in the West generally spend more time sitting than people in the East and are generally taller and heavier in build. Such cultural variations encourage different areas of flexibility and overuse in the body. Because the Thai spend most of their working time in the fields or doing manual labor, their massages focus 75 percent on the lower body and legs. In contrast, westerners spend more time at their desks and computers; the Lotus Palm method consequently focuses equal attention to the lower and upper body.

Throughout this book I will use the term Thai Yoga Massage to describe this healing art and to bring the original principles of Thai massage back to their roots. Part 1 provides the reader with an overview of the fundamental aspects of Thai

Yoga Massage. The theoretical foundations of this healing art will be considered, as will the sen energy lines, the *marma* acupressure points, and the ancient Indian healing system of Ayurveda. Also covered in this section are therapeutic and medical effects of Thai massage, key stances for the practitioner, the importance of meditation in practice, and the spiritual notion of *metta*. In part 2 the reader will be guided through a full-body practice of Thai Yoga Massage. Each posture is fully illustrated for the practitioner, and thoroughly considered in terms of its overall benefits to the receiver.

Enjoy your journey into this dynamic and centering healing dance.

2 Theoretical Foundations
The Sen Lines, the Doshas, and Western Medical Principles

The theoretical roots of most Eastern healing art traditions derive from the philosophy that all forms of life in the universe are animated by an essential life force. In the Indian yoga tradition this energy is called prana, an invisible, silent force that is present in all creation. Prana is extracted from the food we eat, the water we drink, and the air we breathe. It also circulates along a pathway in and around the body, forming a network of vital life force that is essential to the human system. This energy-line theory forms the basis of Thai Yoga Massage.

According to the yoga philosophy upon which Thai Yoga Massage is based, there are 72,000 energy lines running through our *kosha* bodies. The koshas are extensions of the physical body and have five forms or sheaths. The first is the physical body, known as the *annamaya* kosha. The second, the energy body or *pranamaya kosha*, is a layer of life force just above the skin. *Manamaya kosha*, the third layer, is the mental body, where thoughts and doubts are experienced. The fourth is the intellectual body, or *vijnanamaya kosha*, which provides one's identity and sense of self. The fifth is the *anandamaya kosha*, the blissful body that allows one to connect with the metaphysical. Obstruction to the free flow of energy results in an insufficient supply of prana. This could lead to mental, physical, and spiritual imbalances within the kosha bodies, which may be manifested in the form of disease, discomfort, or emotional problems.

Of the 72,000 lines in the Indian tradition, ten are of importance to Thai massage. These lines, known as the *sip sen,* are connected to pressure points (marmas); massaging the sen promotes the free flow of prana. It is through stretching and massaging this network of energy lines that Thai Yoga Massage releases tension, making the entire body more limber. By opening up the body in this way energy flows more easily; this enhanced energy flow helps alleviate common problematic conditions such as lower back pain, arthritis, headaches, digestive difficulties, menstrual problems, and stress-related conditions. Thai Yoga Massage also generates a deep state of relaxation and promotes centeredness and well-being for both the client and the practitioner.

The distinguishing features of Thai Yoga Massage as a bodywork therapy lie in this approach to gently stretching and opening the body.

THE SEN LINES

Many of my students who have studied shiatsu and acupuncture scratch their heads in confusion when studying the sen lines. But, as Confucius says, "Do not be confused!" One of the easiest ways of understanding the Thai sen system is to recognize that it is closely related to the Chinese meridian lines but follows a different medical tradition. While the Chinese system follows the traditional Chinese medicine (TCM) theory that relates energy lines to specific organs, the Thai system, with its foundation in Ayurvedic philosophy, is concerned with the practice of balancing the *tridoshas,* the major elements or building blocks of life, to achieve optimum health. Therefore the emphasis is different.

On the walls of the Wat Pho temple in Bangkok are numerous depictions illustrating the sen lines on the body and specific points along each sen. King Rama III commanded this work of art in 1832, and it still stands today as a foundational source of historic Thai massage knowledge. In 1977 the Association of the Traditional Medical School in Thailand published a book in Thai presenting the medical texts of King Rama III, much of it based on the Wat Pho drawings. In the text, and in the temple, many of the diagrams demonstrating the sen lines are incomplete and the direction of the sen lines unclear. My teacher, Asokananda, and I have spent the past years researching the energy lines as knowledge passed through an unbroken lineage of ancient Thai massage masters. With this research we have been able to identify the key healing properties of the sen lines and continue to map out their pathways on the body.

Following are diagrams depicting the ten sen lines studied in Thai Yoga Massage. The sen lines are shown in gray, and are depicted with both dotted and unbroken lines. Italics indicate that sen's main health indications. The sen lines, and the prana flow through them, can only be detected through experienced intuition; you cannot find the

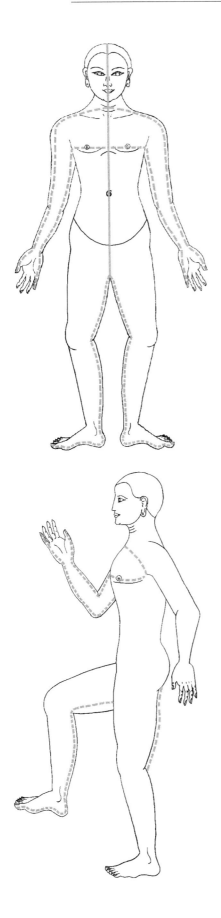

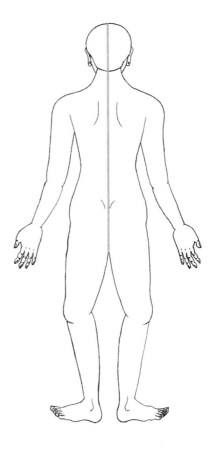

Sen Sumana

Massage to treat *asthma, bronchitis, chest pain*, heart diseases, spasm of the diaphragm, nausea, cold, *cough*, throat problems, diseases of the digestive system, abdominal pain.

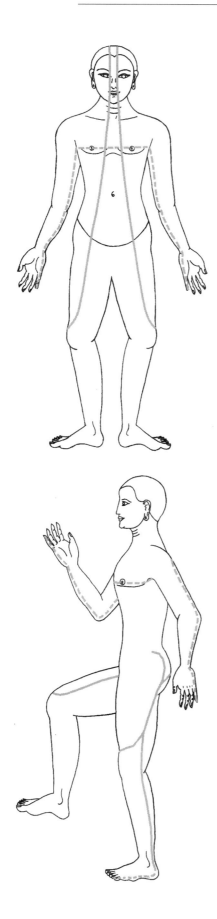

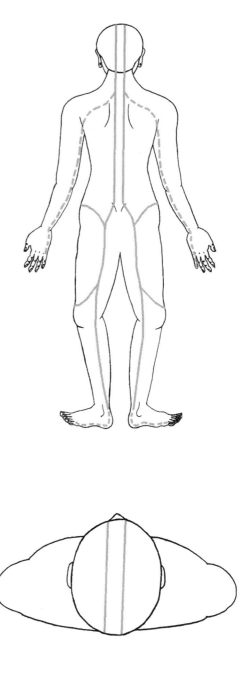

Sen Pingkhala (right side of the body), Sen Ittha (left side of the body)

Massage to treat headache, stiff neck, shoulder pain, common cold, nasal obstruction, throat ache, eye pain, chill and fever, *abdominal pain, intestinal diseases, back pain, diseases of the urinary tract,* dizziness, *diseases of the liver and gallbladder, all internal organs.*

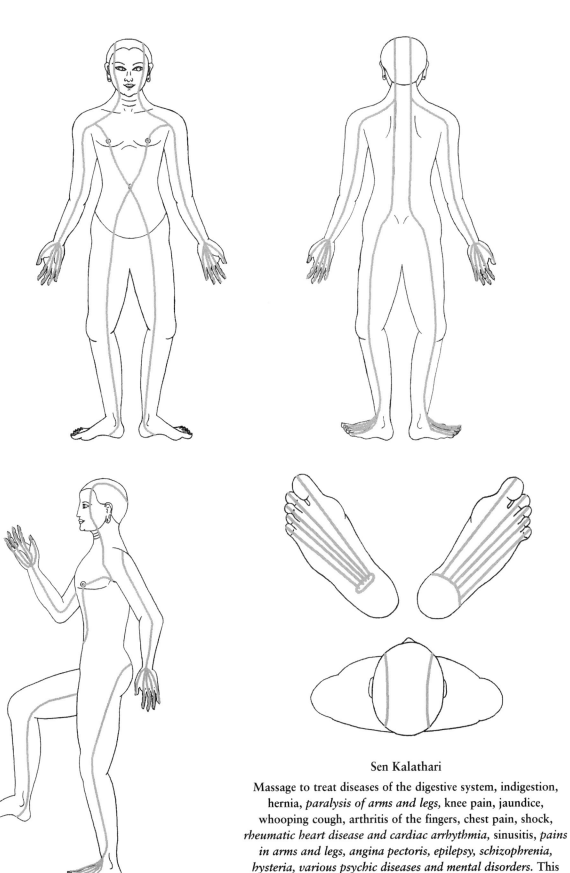

Sen Kalathari

Massage to treat diseases of the digestive system, indigestion, hernia, *paralysis of arms and legs,* knee pain, jaundice, whooping cough, arthritis of the fingers, chest pain, shock, *rheumatic heart disease and cardiac arrhythmia*, sinusitis, *pains in arms and legs, angina pectoris, epilepsy, schizophrenia, hysteria, various psychic diseases and mental disorders*. This line could be called the emotional or psychic line.

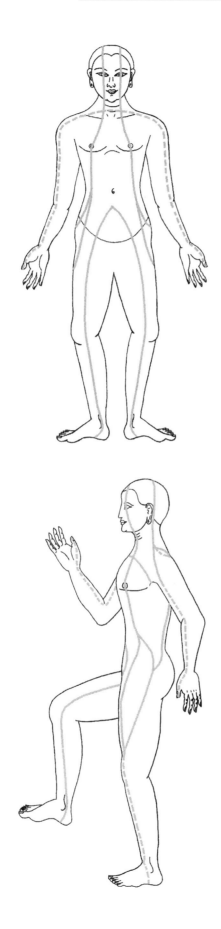

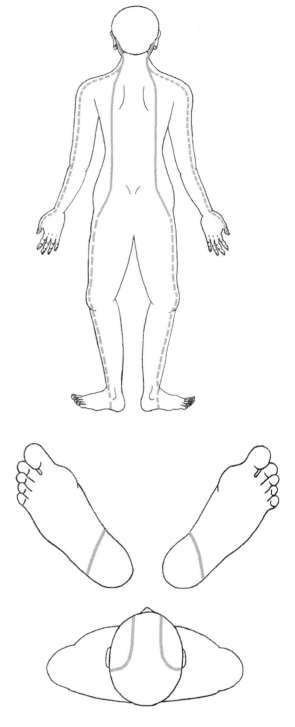

**Sen Thawari (right side of the body),
Sen Sahatsarangsi (left side of the body)**

Massage to treat facial paralysis, toothache, throat ache, redness and swelling of the eye, fever, chest pain, manic-depressive psychosis, gastrointestinal diseases, jaundice, appendix, diseases of the urogenital system, leg paralysis, *arthritis of the knee joint, numbness of lower extremity,* hernia, *knee pain.*

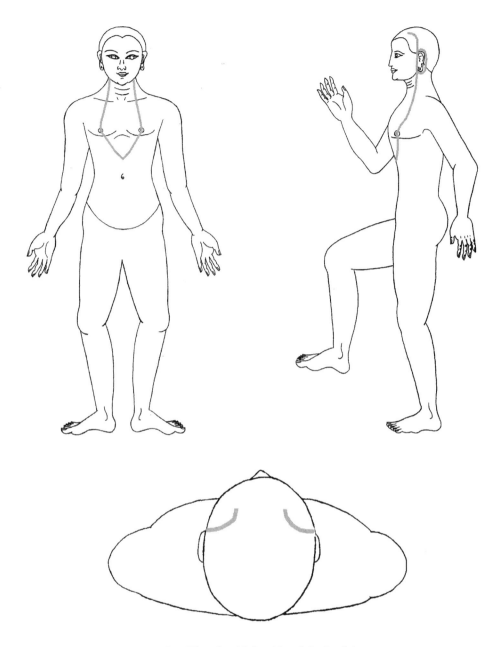

Sen Ulangka (right side of the body),
Sen Lawusang (left side of the body)

Massage to treat *deafness, ear diseases,*
middle ear infections, cough, facial paralysis,
toothache, throat ache, chest pain,
gastrointestinal diseases.

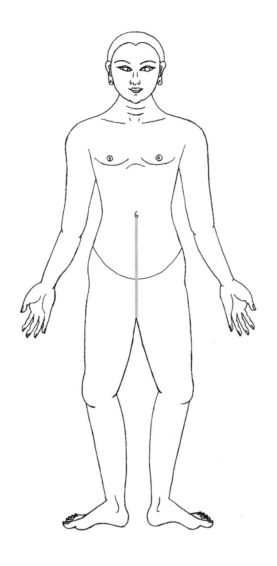

Sen Nanthakrawat, Sen Khitchanna

Sen Nanthakrawat and Sen Khitchanna are generally
worked on by giving an abdominal massage.
Indications are hernia, *frequent urination, female
infertility, impotence, irregular menstruation,
uterine bleeding, retention of urine,*
diarrhea, abdominal pain.

sen lines by dissecting the body. Beginning practitioners often have difficulty sensing the sen. The practice of meditation can help the practitioner develop the skill of feeling the sen by heightening awareness of one's own subtle energies. When the mind is still and concentrated on the present moment, the energy sensations throughout the body become more apparent. The sen anatomical guidelines on the diagrams here and in part two also provide good starting points for further study.

While the sen are not specifically worked in every Thai Yoga Massage movement, they are engaged every time the practitioner palms or thumbs the feet, legs, abdomen, chest, arms and hands, back, and face. The yoga-assisted postures in Thai massage often engage several sen simultaneously. These stretching movements complement the palming and thumbing work, providing a comprehensive bodywork strategy.

MARMAS (PRESSURE POINTS)

Another important element in Ayurvedic massage is the pressure point system of the marmas. Pressure point therapy is an ancient art of healing practiced in many Asian cultures. Along the sen pathway, where the prana flows, are concentrated points, energy centers like spiraling whirlpools that can either retain energy or radiate energy outward. In the Indian tradition these energy centers are called marmas. Often when we fall sick it is because of energy blockages or imbalances in these marmas. Balance and the free flow of prana can be restored by applying pressure to these points, thereby helping to alleviate common ailments, relieve pain, and promote strong energetic flow through the body.

Altogether there are 108 marmas, thirteen are of major significance in Thai Yoga Massage. Seven of these major marma centers are situated along Sen Sumana; these seven marma centers are popularly known as the seven major chakras. The other six marma points—gulpha, zusanli, kshipra, kuprara, amsa, and vidhura marma—can be used in a full bodywork session for general upkeep and to neutralize energy along the sen lines. Each of these marmas has its own specific functions. Gulpha marma, at the feet, relieves stiffness in the ankle joints. Zusanli marma, below the knees, relieves tiredness in the legs. Kshipra marma, at the web of the thumb, relieves tiredness in the hands and arms. Kupara marma, at the inside of the elbows, relieves stiffness in the elbow joints. Amsa marma, on the trapezius, relieves stiffness and soreness on the shoulder, and neck, and vidhura marma, at the base of the skull, relieves headaches.

Thai Yoga Massage works the marmas as part of the sen energy-line circuit. These pressure points are massaged with the practitioner's thumbs, elbows, feet, knees, and other parts of the body.

The therapeutic basis of Thai Yoga Massage is strongly rooted in the Indian healing

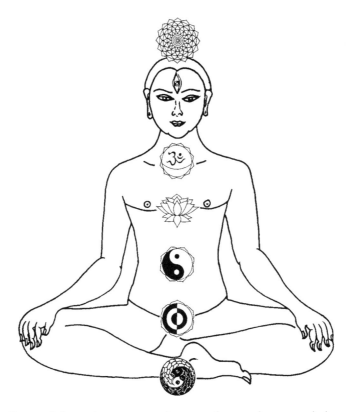

Seven of the major marma points correlate to the seven chakras.

tradition of Ayurveda. The word *ayurveda* derives from two Sanskrit words: *ayur,* meaning "life," and *veda,* meaning "knowledge." Together these words describe a concept of harmonious living; as a body of knowledge, Ayurveda functions as a guide to the proper maintenance of life. The Ayurvedic approach to healing is still practiced in India and Sri Lanka and is now receiving more recognition in the West for its ability to treat the body as a whole. Thai massage developed as an assisted-yoga practice, the rhythm and intensity by which a pose was executed being guided by Ayurvedic principles of constitution: slow and gentle for vata, nonvigorous and relaxing for pitta, energetic and fiery for kapha. Within Thailand the Ayurvedic link to Thai massage has been all but lost; one of the aims of the Lotus Palm method is to bridge the practice of Thai Yoga Massage to its ancient Ayurvedic roots. This does not mean that we intend to operate as Ayurvedic doctors, but rather we integrate some general Ayurvedic principles into our work. This is comparable to shiatsu massage, where practitioners employ the principles of traditional Chinese medicine but are not traditional Chinese medical doctors.

The concepts of Ayurveda introduced here may seem complex, but they will become clearer as you learn and apply them over time.

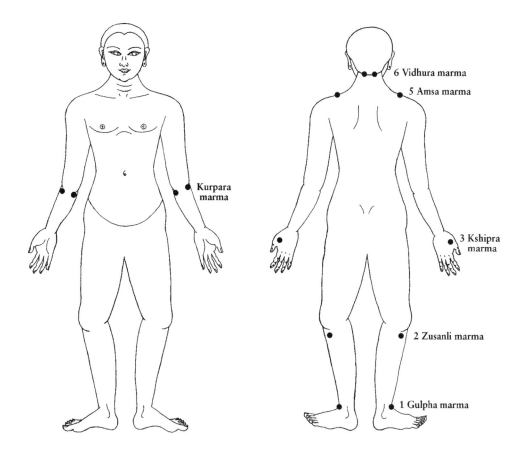

The six special marma points used in a Thai Yoga Massage session

THE FIVE ELEMENTS AND THE TRIDOSHAS

In Ayurvedic philosophy the universe is believed to be composed of five elements, known collectively as the *panchamahabhutas*. These elements are ether, air, fire, water, and earth, and each one is contained in all the others. Let's look at the characteristics of water in studying the five-element phenomenon.

Snow on the ground is an embodiment of water within the principle of the earth element. When the fire element of the sun shines onto the snow, the snow liquefies, forming the characteristic of water. As the heat rises this water evaporates into ether, which later forms clouds, expressing the air principle. These clouds are then condensed into water particles and form rain, returning the principle back to the water element. In this way the five elements of earth, fire, water, ether, and air are represented within the substance of water.

According to Ayurvedic theory, these five elements exist in all matter of the universe, including our own bodies. The five elements are made manifest in the human

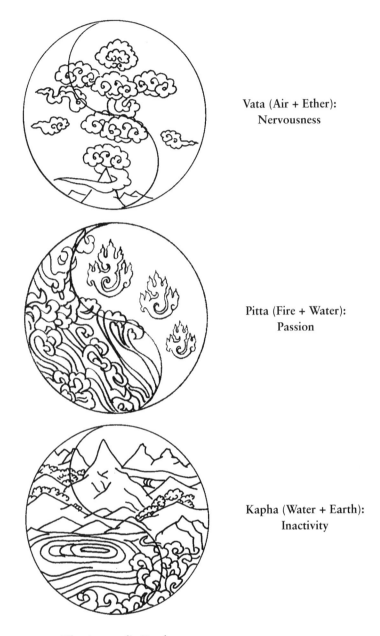

Vata (Air + Ether):
Nervousness

Pitta (Fire + Water):
Passion

Kapha (Water + Earth):
Inactivity

The Ayurvedic Doshas

body in the form of the three Ayurvedic principles known as the *tridoshas*. The ether and air elements combine to form the *vata dosha*, or the air principle. Vata operates within the body to produce movement that relates to the nervous system and the body's energy. The vata dosha is associated with activity, nervousness, agility, and energizing movement. The combination of the fire and water elements within the body form the *pitta dosha,* which is the fire principle that relates to metabolism and diges-tion. The pitta dosha is associated with passion, warmth, circulation, assertiveness, and competition. The elements of earth and water form the *kapha dosha,* the water principle. This dosha is related to the characteristic of water found in the lymph, phlegm, and moisture. The kapha dosha is associated with groundedness, stability, calmness, strength, and consistency.

Ayurvedic medicine aims to achieve optimum health by balancing the doshas of vata, pitta, and kapha through proper diet, exercise, cleansing, meditation, and spiritual and emotional health. This approach can be compared to sending your car to the auto mechanic for a tune-up every now and then. Just as you check your brakes and change your oil, you must regularly tune up the body's functions to maintain an overall good running condition. This is the impetus that brings so many people to a bodywork practitioner. In order to have a healthy and harmonious life it is important to identify the sources of the body's imbalance and methods for achieving equilibrium, the ideal health status being optimal balance in all three doshas. A bodywork practitioner can best begin this study by first understanding his or her own Ayurvedic make-up, and then incorporating into bodywork sessions the knowledge of the Ayurvedic system gained through self-study.

According to Ayurvedic philosophy, each person's natural constitution is made of one or more of the tridoshas. The amount of possible combinations is innumerable, but some general characteristics are unique to each dosha.

Vata Characteristics

Vata people are generally physically small, with protruding veins and bones. They have dark complexions and can be unusually tall or unusually short. They tend to have thin frames, sunken eyes, and coarse hair. Vata people get cold easily and have dry, rough, and cracked skin. They tend to like salty, sweet, and sour foods, as well as hot drinks. They are light sleepers and have restless minds. These people are sensitive, alert, active, and sexually eager. They tire easily and avoid confrontation. Vata people can make money quite easily but will spend it just as quickly. Most diseases in our society are related to an imbalance in vata caused by stress and nervousness.

Pitta Characteristics

Individuals of the pitta nature tend to have medium builds with moderate frames and good muscles. They have reddish complexions with freckles and moist skin, and tend to have fewer wrinkles than vata people. They have thin hair, go prematurely gray, and have hot, sweaty bodies. They usually have big appetites and find it difficult to skip a meal. These detail-oriented people are high achievers. They are passionate; they also have short tempers and may anger easily. Pitta people are leaders in their field and tend to accumulate wealth and material success.

Kapha Characteristics

Kapha people are usually heavy and have stout bodies. They have broad chests and shoulders with well-defined muscles. The kapha complexion is fair and pale. Kapha people have slow digestion and sleep soundly and for many hours. They are generally happy and healthy individuals with good stamina. Kapha people have stable, patient personalities and are slow to anger. They are not easily provoked, but once they are angry it will take them awhile to calm down (I wouldn't stay around when a kapha person gets angry!). They tend to earn a lot of money and are good at retaining their wealth.

AYURVEDA IN THAI YOGA MASSAGE

The Lotus Palm method reconnects Thai Yoga Massage postures with the Indian Ayurvedic principle of the tridoshas. Every time a person is brought into a yoga posture one or all of the doshas is activated; by applying Ayurvedic principles in our work we are able to help balance a recipient's energy and make use of this precious knowledge.

In order to do this the practitioner first uses a questionnaire to identify her client's dosha composition (see the Ayurvedic questionnaire on page 140). Experienced Thai Yoga Massage practitioners will then choose postures to use during the session that will strengthen the recipient's weaker dosha(s). With time this process becomes intuitive. The practitioner also modulates the rhythm and intensity with which she performs the moves, an element of the session that can be just as important as the postures themselves.

Thai yoga postures for vata types
Approach to practice: slow, meditative, gentle, grounded, and
balancing. Postures that build strength, steadiness, stability.

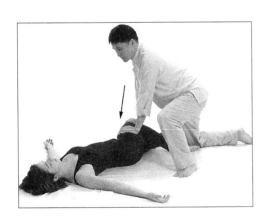

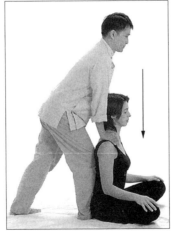

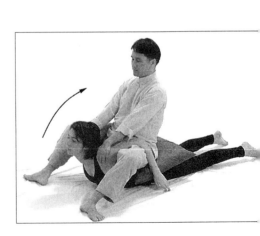

Angel Twist   Palming Shoulders   Pillow Cobra

Thai yoga postures for pitta types

Approach to practice: cooling, relaxing, diffusive, and surrendering. Postures that are nonvigorous, create a cooling effect, and release tension from the mid-abdomen, small intestine, and liver.

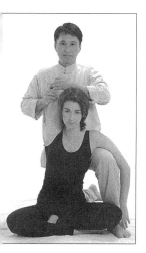

Cow Face 1

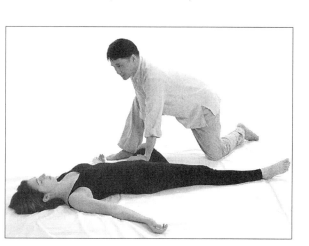

The Tree

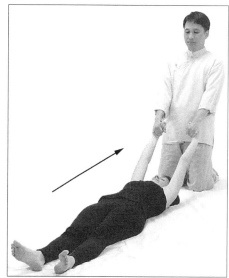

The Long Stretch

Thai yoga postures for kapha types

Approach to practice: fiery, energetic, aerobic, stimulating, and invigorating. Postures that heat up the body, promote circulation of blood, and increase heart capacity.

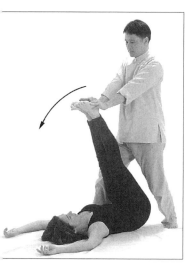

Half-Plough

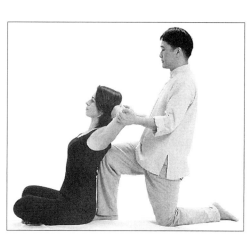

Double Pec Stretch

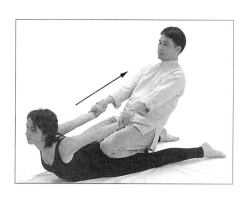

Classic Cobra

Bodywork sessions that are performed slowly, gently, and steadily will reduce vata; those performed with calmness, relaxation, and cooling energy will level out pitta; those practiced with heat, rapid movement, and effort will diminish kapha.

For optimal results a practitioner should approach the entire Thai Yoga Massage session with an understanding of the recipient's constitutional nature. However, the tridoshas are meant to be a general guide, and should be considered among several other factors, such as safety and the receiver's personal preferences. A person should never be forced into a posture that he is uncomfortable with, regardless of whether it is good for his constitution. The specific and immediate needs and requests of the recipient should be addressed first; following that the individual's particular Ayurvedic composition should guide the session.

Each posture in part 2 is accompanied by information on the dosha(s) activated by that posture. The Sun Salutation, a popular series of yoga asanas, provides a good general balancing of all three compositions, as long as the appropriate dosha approach is applied during the practice.

AYURVEDIC CONSTITUTION CHART

	VATA (ACTIVE)	PITTA (PASSIONATE)	KAPHA (SOLID)
Bodyweight	low	moderate	overweight
Frame	thin	moderate	thick
Best approach to life	slow down focusing nurturing gentle discipline via encouragement	calming patience tolerance moderation challenge/lead	energized motivate devote/serve
Recommended diet	cooked: moderate amounts, easily digestible sweet/salty/sour/ oil, (wholesome) moderately spiced	balanced can eat all food in moderation	light and little low-fat, spiced bitter/pungent/ astringent foods
Avoid	raw, heavy, all excesses	spices, coffee, alcohol	dairy fats, rich foods, wheat, oats
Recommended exercise	mild	medium (don't overheat)	vigorous (daily)
Sexual drive	mild	medium	most
Sleep needs	most	medium	least

	VATA (ACTIVE)	PITTA (PASSIONATE)	KAPHA (SOLID)
Recommended work	artistic, intellectual, low stress	leaders, sales, teachers	caretakers, agriculture, nurturing
Health care	gentle and slow, mild dosages	cooling, medium dosages	high dosages slow response,
Best cleansing techniques	enema or herbs/ colon	laxatives/small intestine, liver	fasting head area/ mucus,
Relationship	stay gently warm always	don't overheat, stay out of sun	needs warmth, can do saunas
Best relationships	encouraging	equal/challenging	caretaking
Best massage style	gentle	medium	strong, deep
Vices to avoid	Drugs, sugar, cigarettes, all excesses	Alcohol, ambition	laziness, excess sleep, overeating, greed/hoarding
Recommended yoga postures	slowing/grounding sitting and balancing poses, forward bends	cooling poses with pressure to abdomen (Peacock, Corpse)	vigorous, flowing asanas to boost metabolism (Sun Salutation, Shoulderstand)

WESTERN MEDICAL FOUNDATIONS

More and more these days people seem to be looking for a magic pill to cure sickness, maintain good health, and achieve emotional stability. As most physicians will tell you, exercise and proper hygiene are important elements of a regular health regimen. I, for one, also believe that the "magic" of maintaining good health lies in movement. The body systems stagnate when they aren't pumped and stretched and worked out. As with a pool of water, the various fluids and structural systems that compose the body become stale and ineffective when inert.

While Eastern therapies offer invaluable methods of healing, the accomplishments of Western medicine should not be overlooked in our approach to practice. My wife, who is an emergency doctor, often reminds me of just that! Perhaps the best approach is one that blends the strengths of both worlds to create an integrated perspective. With an understanding of the physiological and anatomical functions of the body, one can better comprehend the benefits and effects of Thai Yoga Massage.

On that note I would like to outline some of the body systems most affected by Thai Yoga Massage.

The Skeletal System

The skeleton is a network of bones that provide the main frame of the body. The skeleton has three major jobs:

1. It gives the body shape.
2. It protects our vital organs, such as the brain, the heart, and the lungs.
3. In partnership with the muscles, it facilitates movement.

The human being is the only animal that walks erect. Keeping upright puts a lot of pressure on the spine as well as on the nonbony structures that support the spine (the tendons, ligaments, and muscles).

The spine is designed to perform six distinct movements: flexion and extension, left and right lateral flexion, and left and right rotation. A Thai Yoga Massage session incorporates these six movements to improve and maintain the health and mobility of the spine. By stretching through various postures, Thai Yoga Massage relieves excess stress in the skeletal body, including the vertebral column. Stretching increases the space between the vertebrae, allowing the lymph, synovial, and cerebrospinal fluids to actively circulate, effectively "greasing" the joints and improving joint mobility. Thai Yoga Massage can correct skeletal problems and even reverse the processes of spinal degeneration diseases such as kyphosis, scoliosis, and lordosis.

When working with the skeletal system you want to avoid putting direct pressure on the bones. Each bone is covered by a sheet of nerves, so it can hurt when bone is touched with too much pressure. As well, it is important to respect the natural range of motion and directional flow of the skeletal joints. Going beyond a joint's range of motion can result in dislocation.

The Circulatory System

The circulatory system is the highway of arteries, veins, and capillaries that connect in a continuous loop, transporting blood, oxygen, and nutrients throughout the body. The heart acts as the pump that keeps this transport system moving. The compression touch technique of palming and thumbing used in Thai Yoga Massage acts as an assistant pump to the heart, increasing the rate of blood flow without causing any strain to the heart. As well, the pressing and pulling of the extremities in Thai Yoga Massage indirectly stimulates local circulatory pathways. Postures that raise the legs higher than the head, such as Half-Plough, Knee to Forehead, and Anti-Gravitational Pose, also encourage the flow of blood back to the heart. The sooner the blood returns to the heart the sooner it begins its journey of delivering blood, oxygen, and nutrients to the body cells and removing waste materials through the venous and lymphatic systems.

Sen Kalathari, the important energy line covering the entire body, runs concurrently with the principal arteries of the body. Palming and thumbing the sen line stimulates the flow of blood in these vessels.

The Muscular System

Muscles are protein tissues composed of cells, or muscle fibers. These fiber bundles are formed in layers that envelop and attach to various bones of the body. Muscles and bones work together as a team. There are more than 600 muscles in the body which together make up at least 40 percent of a person's bodyweight. Muscular activity produces heat, lactic acid, water, and carbon dioxide. These waste products are removed during the process of healthy blood circulation.

Every movement you perform is made possible through the work of muscles. When you eat, sing, run, dance, walk, or practice yoga, it is the muscles that make that action possible. There are two types of muscles within the body: smooth muscles and skeletal muscles. Smooth muscles work automatically and involuntarily; examples of smooth muscles include the stomach, bladder, uterus, and arteries. Skeletal muscles work voluntarily, and are usually attached to bones. Examples of skeletal muscles include the quadriceps, psoas, biceps, and tibialis anterior. Skeletal muscles can also be triggered involuntarily by a "reflex" transmitted through the spinal cord, such as the deep tendon reflex of the knee that causes a person's leg to automatically kick out when the knee is tapped.

The brain, the main power station for muscle activity, sends messages to the body via the spinal cord. Any signal to relax or contract is communicated to the muscles by the body's nervous system. The muscles respond to this signaling process in a yin and yang fashion: a muscle in action (an agonist) is balanced by the work of a muscle stretching in the opposite direction (the antagonist). For example, when you contract your biceps (agonist) you are simultaneously extending your triceps (antagonist). This interdependent relationship—of contracting and simultaneous extending—can be found in all muscles.

In a Thai Yoga Massage session, muscular information can give the practitioner precautionary instructions relative to the postures to be used in the session. For example, the quadriceps and the hamstrings have an agonist/antagonist relationship in many movements, so a strained quadriceps muscle may be further aggravated in a posture such as Snake Creeps Down (see page 96), even though the intention of the posture is to stretch the hamstrings. In this case, the practitioner should use a gentle palming technique to release tension in the quadriceps.

The stretching and massaging in a Thai Yoga Massage session activates the circulation of blood. The mobilization of this important body fluid increases muscular relaxation and elasticity and reduces the effects of adhesions. Thai Yoga Massage also stimulates vascular changes; the mobilization of muscle compresses vessels, affecting the passage of blood and lymph to and from the heart and increasing vascular flow. Stimulating the circulation of blood and lymph helps to eliminate toxins, reducing the risk of thrombosis, edema, and clotting in the vessels.

The Nervous System

The nervous system includes the brain and the spinal cord—the central nervous system—and thousands of myelinated and unmyelinated nerve fibers held together by connective tissue sheaths. Sensory stimuli and motor impulses pass between the brain or other parts of the central nervous system to the muscles, glands, and other parts of the body. The brain is the storehouse and command center for all our bodily actions and functions; the spinal cord is an extension of the brain, sending impulses through and receiving sensory information from the peripheral nerves.

The nervous system breaks down into two categories. The autonomic nervous system regulates involuntary actions, such as the heartbeat, breathing, and digestion, while the somatic nervous system guides sensation and motion. The autonomic nervous system is broken down further into the sympathetic and parasympathetic system. The sympathetic nerves prepare the body for action; the parasympathetic nerves calm the body. The parasympathetic nerves can be considered the agents of "resting and digesting." Thai Yoga Massage stimulates the parasympathetic nervous system, lowering the pulse, slowing the breath, and relaxing the body.

As part of the central nervous system, it is ultimately the brain that oversees the functioning of the entire body, and it is the brain that registers the benefits of tension release. In the spirit of metta (loving-kindness) and the mindfulness of the sacred space that is created in a therapeutic session, Thai Yoga Massage creates a safe, tranquil, healing environment, nurturing the body and encouraging a peaceful bodymind.

3 The Dancing Meditation of Thai Yoga Massage

Many elements that may seem secondary to giving a good massage are of great importance in providing an effective Thai Yoga Massage. A good practitioner is well practiced in the stances and palpation techniques of Thai Yoga Massage and moves in a seamless transition from one posture to the next. This dance of smooth transitions and dynamic movement does not come in one learning session, but with practice your style and comfort will develop.

As you approach this part of your Thai Yoga Massage studies it is good to remember that most movement skills come with easy attention. Grasping toward knowing can result in rigid body use. Remain open and relaxed, and learn with love for yourself. One of the most important practices in learning Thai Yoga Massage—the practice of meditation—will help you let go and ease into the studies in this chapter.

MEDITATION IN THAI YOGA MASSAGE

The role of meditation in Thai Yoga Massage is to assist the practitioner in honing the art of listening, and thus to effectively connect to the recipient and her needs. When there is mindfulness in massage and a spiritual awareness, a sacred healing space is created. In this section, we will consider a few approaches that will help a practitioner to achieve this mindfulness.

Thai massage was originally performed in the Buddhist temples. The masseur approached his job as an extension of his spiritual practice, applying the energy of loving-kindness to the recipient. The masseur's work was a physical application of metta. In Thailand today many massage masters are also great spiritual guides. Masseurs work with full awareness, mindfulness, and concentration and include meditation as part of their daily routine.

Perhaps the most important element in the practice of Thai Yoga Massage is metta, unconditional love and compassion. The notion of metta is not confined to Buddhism; it is a universal principle that can be applied within one's own tradition or belief. My goal as a Thai Yoga Massage teacher is not to have the most famous school but to spread the dharma, the duty, of unconditional love and compassion. There will always be someone practicing a different way of Thai massage, or maybe someone who is better known than you. Real satisfaction in your practice comes from within.

Without some form of spiritual awareness Thai Yoga Massage could become hollow and lose much of its healing power. In my daily practice and in my teaching of Thai Yoga Massage, my students and I open the day with the chant Om mani padme hum, a chant wishing happiness for all beings.

The syllables in this chant have significant meanings. The syllable *Om* refers to the sound vibration that lives within all existence. *Mani* translates as "the jewel"; its extended meaning is about using the sharpness of the jewel to cut through ignorance with wisdom. The word *padme* means "the lotus," symbol of beauty, purity, and compassion that rises and blooms out of a muddy pond. *Hum* is "the open heart," infusing all with kindness and love. The chant is a prayer: "May the jewel in the lotus shine forth this light of love and compassion to unite all existences as one." This chant teaches us that when we bestow kindness on others we actually receive it ourselves.

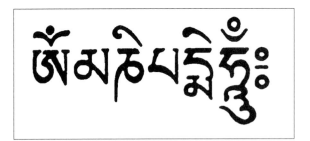

The Tibetan mantra Om Mani Padme Hum

I first became convinced of the power of this chant while traveling by bus from the base of the Himalayan Mountains to the town of Leh in the north of India. The dirt road winds up and down mountains, making for a treacherous journey that can take from three days to one week. Each time the bus driver made a hairpin turn a few of the passengers would chant in unison, "Om mani padme hum."

Upon arriving in Leh I discovered that this magical chant was on the lips of many people I encountered, whether they were cooking, repairing a car, cradling a baby, or simply doing nothing. The place projected a very pleasant and peaceful feeling that I believe is related to the power of this chant and its meaning. For that same benefit Thai Yoga Massage practitioners open the day with this mantra, creating a peaceful, harmonious, and safe atmosphere for working.

In the East there is a saying that "you never step in the same river twice." The water that flows by might look the same, but on closer examination one realizes that it is constantly in flux. This is comparable to life itself—as each moment dies another one is born. In this continuous stream of life, no experience is ever the same as the last.

The practice of meditation helps the Thai Yoga Massage practitioner listen to herself and to the recipient's body from moment to moment. Meditating involves a process of watching the river of consciousness passing by in the mind. Many things may appear in this stream, and the mind will often attach to a subject, allowing it to be carried away along a separate tributary. A little while later another subject may appear and divert our attention, causing us to move in yet another direction. This process continues to repeat itself until, after a while, we end up going in circles. Meanwhile, life is passing us by. By holding on to the past and projecting into the future, we stop living in the present.

Meditation is about being fully alive in this moment—the only reality we can truly know. Meditation teaches us how to be centered and balanced and to detach ourselves from the unnecessary hindrances of life. It reviews the nature of impermanence and gives us the wisdom to live our lives to its fullest.

Being in the present moment is integral to establishing a sacred healing space and being in harmony with the massage. Thai Yoga Massage practitioners take a few moments to empty their thoughts and center themselves at the beginning and end of each session. In the river of life, the breath is the anchor that helps us to focus the wandering mind.

Being mindful of the breath is one of the most useful ways to learn how to meditate. As you inhale, pay attention to your breath and notice the sensation as it enters your nostrils. Feel the cool air as it approaches the back of your throat and notice the fullness of your abdomen. Exhaling, notice the sensations in your belly, lungs, and throat, and the heat at the end of your nostrils as you breathe out.

This form of meditation uses the breath as a point of concentration. As you focus on the sensations of breathing, thoughts of the past and visions of the future are no longer a distraction. If your mind wanders, go back to the breath. This is the soft but focused effort of meditation training, going back to the breath as soon as your mind wanders.

A lot of people think that meditation is about being a sage sitting alone in a cave in the Himalayas. There are some who use meditation to accomplish supernatural feats, but the spirit of meditation in Thai Yoga Massage is about achieving nothing—it is about simply being mindful of the moment. There is a vast difference between a mindful massage and one that is done simply mechanically. In the spirit of mindfulness the practitioner is able to focus more easily on the needs of the recipient, thus respecting the limits of the recipient's body when guiding him into a yoga posture and applying appropriate pressure when palpating. Only through mindfulness can a practitioner develop the skills of listening to the energy flowing through and around the body and feeling the pathways of the sen.

BASIC PRINCIPLES OF MOVEMENT IN THAI YOGA MASSAGE

Thai Yoga Massage is a meditative dance that from moment to moment creates a healing experience. The key to the difference between a good massage and a bad massage is the movement of the practitioner's body. When practitioners use the weight of their bodies rather than brute strength—which can cause discomfort to the recipient and fatigue for the practitioner—recipients have the full benefit of a consistent, rhythmic pressure that is deeply relaxing. For practitioners, long-established poor habits in movement can cause back pain, tendinitis, stiff neck, and other conditions, and can eventually force an individual to give up his practice.

My first time teaching outside of Thailand was in Edenkoben, a small town in southwest Germany. I was invited to do a presentation on the art of Thai Yoga Massage in a school of traditional Western massage therapy. The school's directors invited me because they had seen pictures of Thai massage and could not resist its beautiful esthetic. I was forewarned, however, that the students could be skeptical about Eastern methods of healing based on the concept of prana, or energy flow.

When I entered the lecture room I was greeted by forty people in groups of four or five. Group leaders, who were surrounded by skeletons and charts, pointed out different parts of the body while the others listened. Everyone would join together in a unison chant, naming the different parts of the body. At this point I sensed that any one of these individuals knew the anatomy of the body better than most massage masters in the East. It dawned on me how little Eastern bodyworkers actually know about the body in terms of its structural and physiological functions.

I began my presentation with an introduction to the history, theory, and spiritual aspects of Thai Yoga Massage. The second part of my presentation was a sped-up demonstration of how to perform Thai Yoga Massage, and the third part was hands-on massage practice using the Thai Yoga Massage techniques.

It was during the third part of my presentation that I realized this group could learn something valuable from Eastern practices. While the students I was teaching had been trained to identify all the different parts of the body, they were never taught how to use their own bodies effectively. This was one of the most awkward groups of practitioners I had ever encountered. They were off-center, and their movements were anything but graceful.

In the East, Thai massage practitioners place a lot of importance on the dance of the massage. Principles of fluid movement and body centering are key elements of Thai Yoga Massage. I have cultivated a movement style with stances inspired by the Chinese martial art of tai chi chuan as an especially important element in linking postures in a Thai Yoga Massage session. The way of listening with one's whole being that is the hallmark of the tai chi chuan art of pushing hands is the same kind of attentiveness that must be cultivated in order to practice Thai Yoga Massage. In this way, a martial art is transformed into a healing art.

In Edenkoben, a presentation that began with a great amount of curiosity (and skepticism) ended in great enthusiasm. The response from this group of professional students was very encouraging. They recognized the dance in Thai Yoga Massage and realized that effective massage actually begins with the practitioner's own body awareness.

THE RHYTHMIC ROCKING DANCE

The essential movement within Thai Yoga Massage is the rhythmic rocking dance. This technique involves the practitioner swaying his body in a rocking motion such that his bodyweight creates a natural and even pressure on the recipient's body. With straight arms and a straight spine, the practitioner moves back and forth in a swaying rhythm that resembles the movement of a bamboo reed. The pacing is repetitive but not overly mechanical. The practitioner embodies the smoothness of a cat as it walks, the motion gently rocking the recipient's body, as if cradling a baby to sleep. This sedative dance sets the pace for the entire bodywork session.

The movement of the rhythmic rocking dance is like a tai chi meditation sequence; you learn how to play with the circular energy of chi, and to use the least amount of effort to achieve maximum results. When we hear the word *massage* we usually think of using our hands and thumbs to squeeze muscles. But if you know how to use your whole body in the rhythmic rocking dance when giving a massage, you can conserve energy and avoid becoming exhausted. You can also prevent the development of chronic stress syndromes in the hands, arms, and shoulders.

Instead of using your muscles, the rhythmic rocking dance maximizes your energy by allowing it to circulate down the spine. The energy is then centered on the second chakra—the swadhisthana chakra, the space three fingers below your belly button—and flows into your arms and palms. When you dance this dance successfully you actually borrow energy from the earth. This way, even when you apply a good amount of pressure in the course of a session, you do not feel tired at the end of the massage.

The rhythmic rocking dance is the base for three floor techniques used in working with clients; those techniques are the bamboo (side) rock, the forward rock, and the whirlpool or circular rock.

Bamboo Rock (Side Rock)

In the bamboo rock the practitioner kneels, knees spread or pressed together and the tops of the feet on the mat forming a solid base. Tuck the chin in slightly to straighten the spine; the alignment from crown to coccyx should be pure, yet relaxed. Straighten your arms and shift the trunk of the body from side to side, swaying the torso like a bamboo in the wind.

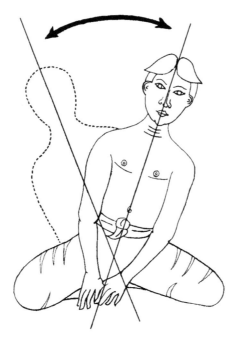

Bamboo Rock (Side Rock)

Forward Rock

In the forward rock the practitioner begins again by kneeling, knees spread or pressed together and the tops of the feet on the mat forming a solid base. Tuck the chin in slightly, straightening the spine. The alignment from crown to coccyx is straight but relaxed. Maintaining this alignment, rock the torso forward and backward, like a rocking chair.

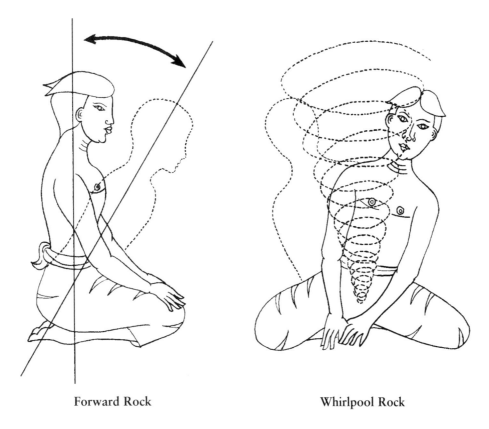

Forward Rock   Whirlpool Rock

Whirlpool Rock (Circular Rock)

In the whirlpool rock the practitioner begins as above: knees spread or pressed together and the tops of the feet on the mat forming a solid base. Tuck the chin in slightly to straighten the spine; maintain a strong yet relaxed alignment from crown to coccyx. Keeping this alignment, circulate the torso clockwise or counterclockwise in a whirlpool motion, using the coccyx as the axis. Be sure to circulate the entire torso.

—⚏—

The practitioner applies one of these rocking techniques at a time. The rhythm created by the rocking techniques can be compared to the tempo underlying any musical score; this pace is always present and provides the structure for the entire session. In many ways the success of a Thai Yoga Massage session, both for the receiver and the giver, is closely linked to the proper application of the three rocking techniques.

The postures in part 2 include recommendations as to which rocking technique is best to use in each posture. After practicing for some time, allow your intuition to guide your movement in the rhythmic rocking dance.

THE WORKING STANCES

Thai Yoga Massage is a beautiful dance that requires continuous movement by the practitioner to provide a relaxed and flowing session for the recipient. It is therefore extremely important that the practitioner uses his body well, moving with effortless, graceful transitions. Ancient lessons of fluid movement and proper body mechanics are extracted from the traditions of tai chi and yoga as a foundation for the working stances described below.

When holding a working stance within Thai Yoga Massage, consider the tree as inspiration for your position. Imagine your arms and hands are the branches, strong yet yielding. They are connected to your spine, which is the trunk of a tree, sturdy and erect. The spine transfers your body's weight to your feet, which are the roots, firmly planted in the earth. By keeping your spine straight and your head up, you are aligning the seven energy centers (the chakras) along the spine. Combining the energy of earth and heaven, like the tree, with the energy of your body, you maintain a strong yet resilient posture that is fluid in every aspect of its movement.

A common mistake for bodywork practitioners is hunching through the back and losing strong spinal alignment through the course of a session. When the body is hunched over in this way, the practitioner is using her shoulders instead of connecting her body to the earth. This position can result in a sore back and fatigue for the practitioner, and a less-than-effective massage for the recipient. Always keep the image of the tree present in your body as you practice these stances.

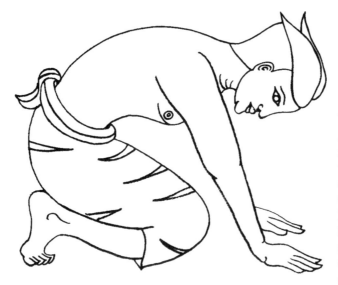

When holding a Thai Yoga Massage working stance, it is most important to maintain the structural integrity of the spine, and the alignment of the chakras along the spine. Rounding the shoulders and hunching over the recipient results in fatigue and an unsatisfactory massage experience.

The three rocking techniques of bamboo rock, forward rock, and whirlpool rock can be applied with any of the stances described below. When applying pressure that alternates from side to side, use the bamboo rock; for frontward movement or pressure, use the forward rock; and for any circular techniques, use the whirlpool rock.

Diamond Stance

Kneel on the mat with your knees together, buttocks resting on your heels. The tops of your feet are flat on the mat.

Open Diamond

Kneel on the mat with your knees spread apart and your buttocks resting on your heels. The tops of your feet are flat on the mat.

Kneeling Diamond

Stand up on your knees, your body forming a plane from your knees to the crown of your head. Tuck your tailbone slightly and keep your back erect.

Cat 1

Kneel on the mat with your knees spread, buttocks resting on your heels and the tops of your feet on the ground. Hinge forward slightly from the hips and place your palms

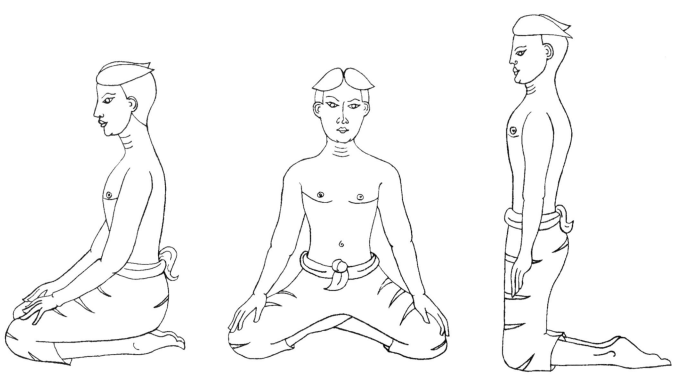

Diamond Stance   Open Diamond   Kneeling Diamond

flat on the mat. Keep your arms and back straight. Practice the bamboo rock: move from your second chakra and press alternating palms onto the mat.

Cat 2

Kneel on the mat with your knees spread, buttocks resting on your heels and your toes curled under, providing a lift under your buttocks. Hinge forward slightly from your hips and place your palms flat on the mat, keeping your arms and back straight. Practice the bamboo rock, moving from your second chakra and pressing alternating palms onto the mat.

Cat 3

Kneel on all fours with your knees under your hips. In yoga this is sometimes called the Tabletop. Keep your back and arms straight. Practice the bamboo rock: move from your second chakra and press alternating palms onto the mat.

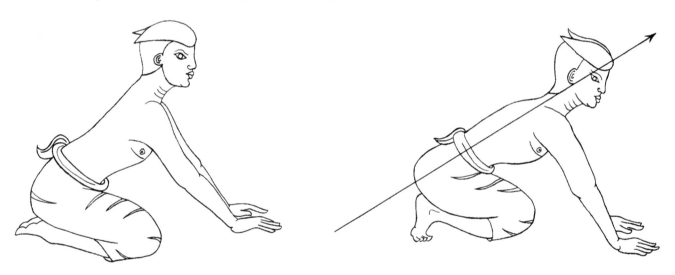

Cat 1   Cat 2

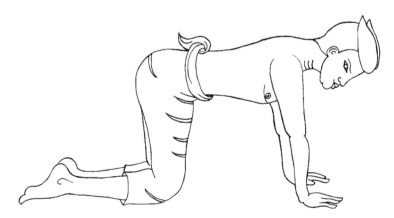

Cat 3

Warrior Stance

From the Kneeling Diamond stance (see page 35), rise up on one knee. Keep your arms and back straight. Move from the second chakra as you work on the recipient. Be careful that the raised knee does not extend beyond the toes; the front heel is grounded. This is the most frequently used stance in a Thai Yoga Massage session.

Archer Stance

In a squatting stance, the toes of both feet are tucked under. Place one knee on the ground. Keep your back straight. This is a tricky pose, requiring strength and balance. Practice, practice, practice.

Tai Chi Stance

Stand with feet shoulder-width apart; legs are straight but knees are soft. Step forward a comfortable distance, straightening your back leg and bending your front knee slightly. Do not let your bent knee extend past your toes. The front foot is pointing directly ahead and the back foot is naturally turned outward. Maintain a stable center, with 70 percent of your weight on the front leg and 30 percent on the back leg.

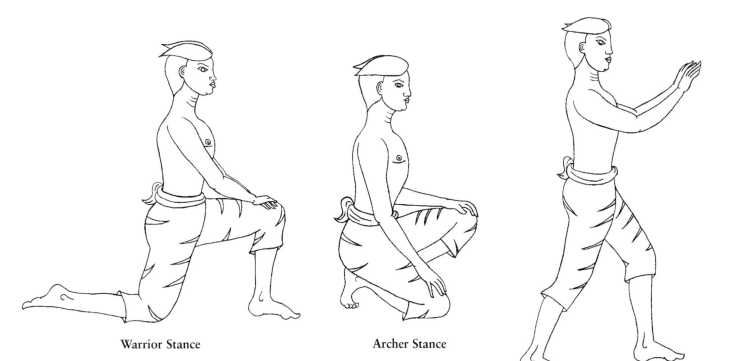

Warrior Stance   Archer Stance

Tai Chi Stance

—⚍—

Thai Yoga Massage is a very physical form of therapy—a treatment, which typically takes one to two hours, is often an athletic workout for the practitioner. Keeping this in mind, the proper use of the practitioner's body weight should not be replaced with muscular strength. Frequently the muscles of the hand and the upper shoulder are overused; practitioners commonly make the mistake of bending the arms, curving the back, and tilting the head downward. While this kind of a posture may feel more natural than the stances described above, it actually disconnects the upper body from the lower body, leading to weakened rapport with the recipient. A practitioner's poor posture can interrupt his state of meditative awareness and encourage fatigue. The proper use of body weight ensures constant pressure, which is comforting to the recipient's nervous system and adds positive effects overall to the massage session.

In traditional Chinese medicine, the three energies of earth, heaven, and body are called the three treasures. They are made manifest in our bodies as ching, the energy we are born with; chi, the energy of life force; and shen, the energy of inner heart or spirit. By physically aligning the body in the working stances described here, we allow these three treasures to unite. That unity provides strength to our bodywork session.

TOUCH TECHNIQUES

The manipulations that are most frequently employed in Thai Yoga Massage are the techniques of palming and thumbing. Palming is generally used to open and warm up the body and stimulate the energy lines before beginning the technique of thumbing.

Palming

In palming, the practitioner uses the area of the palm close to the heel of the hand to compress the energy lines of the recipient's body. You must not use the heel of the hand exclusively, as this could feel like a stick poking into the recipient's body. When palming, cup your hands with your fingers slightly spread, as if you're holding on to a basketball. Be careful not to overflex your wrist, as this could lead to injuries over time. Keep your arms and back straight but not rigid; your head is aligned on your spine. From this position, "fall in" to the recipient's body with your weight, using bamboo rock or forward rock.

Thumbing

Thumbing is a technique that can best be described as thumb chasing thumb. Using her bodyweight, the practitioner uses the bamboo or forward rock to press her thumbs into the recipient's body. As with palming, the practitioner keeps arms and spine straight.

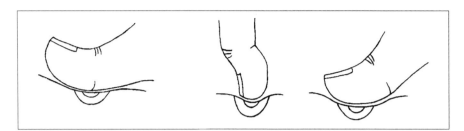

Incorrect (left): Hyperextension can lead to thumb injury.
Incorrect (center): Applying pressure with the tip of the thumb can cause discomfort for the recipient.
Correct (right): Use the pad of the thumb when applying pressure in thumbing.

This sets up a supportive posture for using the thumbs sensibly, an essential element in avoiding overuse injuries as well as providing the most comfort to the recipient.

The correct method for thumbing is to use the pad of the thumb; common mistakes are hyperextending the thumb or pressing the thumbnail into the recipient.

—m—

Thai Yoga Massage encourages the use of other body parts as tools for the massage. Besides the techniques of palming and thumbing, the forearms, elbows, knees, and feet can be useful as well.

Forearms

The forearms are used for smoothing and rolling the muscles in preparation for deep-pressure work on the recipient's body. The practitioner places the forearm on the recipient's body, gradually rocking in with the body's weight as the forearm rolls away from the practitionet. Take care not to use the bony part of the forearm close to the elbow; the ulna bone can be sharp and produce an unpleasant feeling in the recipient.

Elbows

Elbows are very effective tools if the recipient requests deeper pressure. The elbows are used to apply direct pressure on a specific part of the body. Place the elbow on the recipient's body and, with a relaxed shoulder and upper body, gradually lean in with your bodyweight. To prevent the elbow from slipping you can hook the thumb and forefinger of the opposite hand around the elbow. Continue using the hand as a guide along the recipient's body.

Knees

The knees can produce an even more powerful effect upon the recipient's body than the elbows. The use of the knees demands good balance and agility on the part of the practitioner.

Positioning your hands on the recipient as support, place the knees on the recipient's body. Gradually lean in with your bodyweight—sparingly, as the appropriate amount of pressure is difficult to judge.

Feet

The feet have many nerve endings, enabling them to be as responsive as the hand in giving and receiving information. The feet can be used for applying direct pressure, as well as for stabilizing the recipient in postures and stretches. The numerous parts of the foot—the heel, instep, blade of the foot, dorsal, ball of the foot, and toes can be used in countless ways in the massage. The foot is as versatile as the hand; this should be kept in mind when practicing. Specific examples of using the feet for massage are given in the posture instructions in part 2.

BREATHING TECHNIQUES IN THAI YOGA MASSAGE

Breath and movement are synonymous. Thai Yoga Massage is a dynamic form of bodywork; it is a shared choreography of palming, postures, and body placement. Within the Lotus Palm method of Thai Yoga Massage we teach four breath techniques to increase the benefit of our practice, both for the recipient and the practitioner.

Mindful Breathing

Mindful breath is closely associated with the meditative state in Thai Yoga Massage. Mindful breath is a meditation in motion, with the practitioner observing his breath from moment to moment as the dance of the massage unfolds. In this way the practitioner is fully focused on the work with the recipient. Mindful breathing is the most commonly used breath technique in a Thai Yoga Massage session.

Synchronized Breathing

In synchronized breathing the practitioner is attentive to the recipient's breath and mimics its rhythm. This technique is mainly used when massaging the abdominal region. This tender area of the body houses many of our vital organs. When the practitioner marries a therapeutic touch with the breath, the result can be a very soothing, calming experience.

Directed Breathing

With directed breathing the practitioner indicates to the recipient when to inhale and when to exhale, the breath matching different stages of a posture or stretch. For example, in the Cobra posture (see page 115) the practitioner asks the recipient to inhale

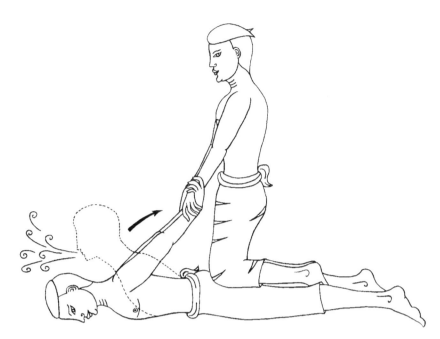

Proper breathing is essential to the release of physical and mental tension in all Thai Yoga Massage postures. In this depiction of directed breathing the recipient is guided to exhale when placed into the Cobra, as the dotted figure demonstrates.

while still on the ground, and then directs the recipient to exhale as he is assisted into the Cobra pose. This technique is useful in enabling the practitioner to give the recipient a deeper stretch, and generally results in a good release of tension from the body.

Induced Breathing

When practicing induced breathing the practitioner follows the recipient's exhalation and then gradually applies pressure to the body, forcing a deeper release of the breath. This technique is mainly used while working on the back, an area of the body that can hold a lot of tension. Awareness of the breath is not always evident in the back; a forceful exhalation brings an inhalation full of awareness to any area of the back that has been compressed. This encourages a great release of tension. It is very comforting to remain passive as a recipient and be brought to a breath in this way.

—⁓—

There are a few points to bear in mind when practicing breath technique in Thai Yoga Massage. It can be intrusive for the practitioner to overmanipulate the recipient's breath. Likewise, strong, noisy breathing, as if somebody is breathing close to the ear, can disturb the recipient's state of rest. In this situation the recipient can be misled to synchronize with the practitioner's breath when that is unnecessary. Keep in mind that in a Thai Yoga Massage session the recipient is in a passive state and the practitioner is active, producing a very different breath rhythm for each. As well, each person's lung capacity is different. Don't feel that you are in a rush during a session and go chasing after the recipient's breath. Staying mindful will allow a gentle rhythm to emerge between you.

STAYING CONNECTED

Continually applying metta, loving-kindness, will keep you connected with the recipient and aware of the recipient's response to the firm pressure and deep stretches of Thai Yoga Massage. My students often ask me how much pressure should be applied during the bodywork session. The best gauge is to start off with a gradual application of one's bodyweight and then ask the recipient for feedback.

In a Thai Yoga Massage session, the rhythmic rocking dance evens out the energy released in the practitioner's body during palming, thumbing, and forearm or foot massage. Yet, while developing a sense of self-awareness and movement as a practitioner is integral to successful practice of Thai Yoga Massage, it should not overshadow the importance of being attentive to the recipient. Keep a close rapport with the recipient throughout the session by constantly watching for changes in facial expressions and muscle tension. Oftentimes recipients will not tell you how much pressure is too much. In general, the way the body is feeling is communicated through the face. If the recipient cringes, be sure to reduce your massage pressure or the extent of the stretch.

Here are four points that may help you stay focused on the needs of the person to whom you are giving a Thai Yoga Massage session.

- Maintain the meditative openness of moment-to-moment awareness.
- Cultivate contact with your recipient by "listening" with your hands and body, keeping regular eye contact, and paying attention to your intuition.
- Respect the recipient's physical, emotional, and sexual boundaries. Synchronize your breathing with the work and be aware of the recipient's breathing.
- Uphold the tradition of Thai Yoga Massage by basing your practice on loving-kindness and compassion.

An important element to the Ayurvedic approach of Thai Yoga Massage is the philosophy of self-care. As a follow-up to each session, the practitioner well studied in Ayurveda recommends diet, exercises, yoga postures, and meditation for her client to practice at home before the next session. I encourage developing a progressive treatment plan that builds on each session and promotes a relationship between the practitioner and client. At the end of a session it is always good to ask the recipient which positions she prefers or dislikes, so that you are aware for the next time. You might recommend that the recipient return every two weeks to maintain her bodywork therapy.

In the Eastern tradition of healing it is the responsibility of the practitioner to keep his client in good health. In fact, custom in the East holds that you do not get paid if your client is sick. So good luck to you!

4 The Practitioner/Client Relationship

Thai Yoga Massage is a vigorous form of massage that uses a lot of physical maneuvers. It involves spinal movements, stretching of the joints and muscles, and placing the recipient in a series of yoga postures. Since the spine contains the main telecommunication system of all the major bodily functions, it is extremely important to practice Thai Yoga Massage with great care and attention. While it is important to perform the postures properly and safely to have the full beneficial effect, we must always respect the recipient's physical limitations and emotional boundaries. Postures not performed in a proper manner can have a deleterious effect, such as creating musculoskeletal imbalances and constricting muscles.

Here are a few pointers for practicing safe massage.

1. Always begin your first session with a recipient by having him complete the health questionnaire on page 137. Ask the recipient about the state of his health and any physical limitations and fears of injury he may have. If you don't understand any medical terms used, ask for further explanation; when in doubt, ask the recipient to get prior approval for Thai Yoga Massage from a health practitioner. Place the questionnaire close by so you can refer to it easily while giving the massage.

2. Don't use force or jerky movements. When placing the recipient in a Thai yoga

posture or making a transition from one position to another, use your body-weight rather than muscular force. Keep your arms, back, and head aligned, and your hands relaxed. Proper alignment facilitates smoother, continuous movement. Ask the recipient to give you feedback if any discomfort is experienced, or if he reaches his limit when receiving a stretch or pressure.

3. Keep safe stances. Center yourself from the second chakra, the swadhisthana chakra, three fingers below the navel. Keep your spine straight and your head properly aligned with your spine at all times, bearing in mind that you need a solid base to work from. A solid stance helps prevent clumsiness that might result in a false move or a fall. And, in the long run, a solid stance is better for your back.

4. Maintain proper alignment. Thai Yoga Massage is a dynamic form of massage that involves placing the recipient in various positions. If you are not careful the recipient can end up spread out in an awkward and twisted manner. Use props and pillows to correctly align the recipient when you need to.

5. Follow the natural anatomical flow of the recipient's body. In all my years of teaching not one of my students has twisted a finger or displaced a bone (thanks, Buddha!). Do not put pressure on joints and bones. It is important to have a sound knowledge of body mechanics as a basis for a safe Thai Yoga Massage practice.

6. Do the dance. Move in a fluid manner, using the rhythmic rocking techniques described on pages 31–33. The dance in Thai Yoga Massage is the basis for an elegant and economic use of energy and helps prevent a build-up of tension or fatigue. When you employ the dance of Thai Yoga Massage, the recipient feels the benefit of your full presence.

7. Monkey see, monkey do. As a beginning practitioner it is wise to follow the form that is being taught rather than innovating right at the start. This is not to curb your creativity but rather to help you consolidate the basic form, perfect the nuances, and understand the work thoroughly.

8. Follow standard rules of personal hygiene. Wash your hands before and after a massage. Keep your fingernails (and toenails) trimmed and clean. If the recipient indicates that he has a skin problem, find out whether it is contagious before beginning the massage; avoid working on open wounds or areas affected by recent surgery or injuries. It is always better to err on the side of safety and precaution. Wear clean, comfortable clothes that fit properly. Keep your massage area clean; do the same with any sheets, blankets, or pillows that you use.

9. Keeping your recipient safe is one thing; keeping yourself safe is another. A ten-minute routine to limber up, especially around the wrists and hips, before commencing a massage can save you from injury.

10. Respect universally accepted sexual boundaries. Use a pillow to create a boundary between you and the recipient for positions that involve close body-to-body contact. When massaging the abdomen and chest don't climb over the recipient's body or straddle it in a Warrior stance. Avoid the breast and genital areas. The recipient should always feel safe and respected—use common sense, and err on the side of caution.

A good carpenter relies on good tools; the same goes for a good Thai Yoga Massage practitioner. Although it is not traditionally Thai, the use of props and pillows gives extra comfort and supports the recipient's alignment, thus creating a better working environment for the practitioner. One must not forget the importance of the ambience of the massage room either. It is essential to keep the room clean and neat, and to check that the recipient is comfortable with the room temperature. Having plants and adequate sunlight makes it more pleasant. However, making do without props is also an important skill to acquire in learning how to integrate the basic *do*'s and *don't*s of Thai Yoga Massage in a creative and resourceful way. I myself have practiced massage in the most unimaginable places, often under difficult circumstances.

How does a practitioner deal with a recipient's emotional release? While we must acknowledge that we are not psychotherapists, we cannot ignore the fact that massage has a psychological and emotional impact. According to yoga philosophy, a bodyworker is in contact with a person's five energy bodies, or sheaths: the physical sheath, the energy sheath, the mental sheath, the intellectual sheath, and the blissful sheath. Because a Thai Yoga Massage experience touches on each of these aspects of a person, buried emotional issues may sometimes surface and trigger an emotional release.

Once while working on a student at a workshop in Austria I noticed a smell that was neither sweet nor foul, but something I could not name. As it turned out, what I smelled was trouble. Toward the end of the massage the student's body started shaking and then bouncing up and down. She cried out for her mother and father and began screaming until she was hoarse. This went on for a while—for how long, I don't know, but long enough for people to come and peer through the window.

What could I do? I decided to sit next to her in a meditation pose to provide the space for this disturbing energy to dissipate. She continued wailing and screaming for so long that I lost track of time. For one moment I felt like wailing and screaming myself, as if the energy had shifted over to me. Yet all the meditation I had practiced did not go to waste, and it enabled me to be there and let go at the same time.

After a while the woman gave me a hug and fell asleep. On my way out I saw some crystals lying on the windowsill with incense, Tibetan bells, and other purifying agents. Maybe out of superstition, or else just to be on the safe side, I picked up a crystal and started clearing my energy field and that of the people dearest to me. That night I slept well.

The next morning, lo and behold, the first person I met was that same student! She gave me another big hug and thanked me for being there. The smell was still present, but it was greatly diminished from the day before.

I returned to Vienna to give a workshop one year later. I was again booked to do a session with the same student. With a concerned expression on her face the organizer asked, "Do you want to give this massage? This time it is at her house." As a warrior, I would never pass up a challenge like that.

I knocked on the student's door and she greeted me with a welcoming hug. I recognized the acrid smell right away, but it was now masked by the aromatherapy scent within her house. On her walls were pictures and paintings of people from all over the world and through time—an Indian mystic, warriors, older women, young women. I had no doubt that the student was communicating with these images.

Just before putting on my massage clothes the woman insisted that I change into something white.

The massage went well but, as before, the student went into convulsions, this time without screaming. It was as if another being was inside her, coming out in movements. Some of the movements constricted her spine and others resembled yoga postures. I sat down and meditated. This went on for a while. Eventually the woman rested beside me as I sat meditating.

After lying down for a while, she cooked me a good meal and off I went, until the next time.

Thai Yoga Massage practitioners should practice metta, loving compassion, and neither encourage nor discourage emotional release. It is important to be fully present for the recipient and not avoid issues or be caught unprepared. Simply pause and allow the emotional release to pass. This is where the practice of vipassana, open observation, comes in handy, helping the practitioner create space for such energy to move and dissipate. Vipassana also reminds us of the impermanence of all things. The practitioner's role is to "note and let go."

CONTRAINDICATIONS

While massage to most areas of the body is beneficial at most times, there are circumstances in which the massage should be modified or altogether avoided. Contraindications are situations in which massage could aggravate or jeopardize the health problem of your recipient. In some cases, massage may be possible if the practitioner stays away from the problematic area.

As practitioners of Thai Yoga Massage, we should be informed of all the recipient's health problems and attain some introductory knowledge of certain diseases and their causes. This will allow us to approach our work effectively with great caution and safety. The brief descriptives here will give you a starting point for ways to approach various health conditions. Further information may be necessary for you to feel grounded in your treatment of specific people.

AIDS

AIDS is the syndrome resulting from infection by the human immunodeficiency virus (HIV). The disease causes the immune system to weaken. People with AIDS are prone to cancer and infection.

Precaution: If you have a contagious condition, such as herpes or a head cold, do not massage a person with AIDS. Since AIDS is only transmitted through blood and body secretions, there is no reason to refuse a client with AIDS if you follow universal precautions.

Allergies

An allergy is an acquired hypersensitivity to a substance.

Precaution: Make sure the recipient is not allergic to aromatherapeutic oils that you might apply at the end of the session. Ask before burning incense. Keep pets away from the recipient.

Aneurysm

Aneurysms can occur in virtually any artery of the body, but the brain, chest, and abdomen are the most frequent sites of fatal aneurysm. Aneurysm is a disease of the arteries that may occur when one has arteriosclerosis. An aneurysm is a localized, blood-filled dilation of a blood vessel caused by disease or weakening of the vessel wall.

Precaution: If the recipient has an abdominal aortic aneurysm, do not press on her abdomen. In the case of a brain or thoracic aneurysm, obviously one cannot dangerously compress the skull or thorax. However, it would be safer, especially in the case of a brain aneurysm, to avoid any inverted exercises or postures that block respiration, thereby increasing blood pressure to the brain.

Arteriosclerosis

Arteriosclerosis is a thickening of the walls of the arteries that leads to impaired blood circulation. When the walls of the arteries thicken they become "plugged," obstructing blood circulation to the heart and potentially leading to heart disease. Arteriosclerosis can also affect the brain vessels and lead to a stroke. The condition can be caused by elevated cholesterol. Because blood is the main provider of the body's nutrients and oxygen, arteriosclerosis has the potential to be quite damaging to the body.

Precaution: Avoid inverted postures, compressing in one area for too long, and pressing on the principle arteries—the carotid arteries on the neck, the femoral arteries on the pelvis, and the brachial arteries near the armpits.

Articulation Disorders

Articulation disorders, otherwise known as joint problems, include any instability in the joints due to damage to the ligaments, menisci, synovial bursae, and bones. Examples of articulation disorders include gouty arthritis, menisci tear, knee sprain, and ankle sprain.

Precaution: Go easy when massaging the affected joint. Never put pressure on the problem area.

Cancer

Cancer is a growth of abnormal cells that can spread to all parts of the body. If the cancer has affected the bones they become fragile and can easily break.

Precaution: The precautions for working with a recipient with cancer are the same as for osteoporosis; avoid brisk movements and applying too much direct pressure. Be especially careful when working on the cervical spine and chest of a person with cancer. Do not work on clients with lymphatic cancer. In all cases of cancer, consult a licensed health practitioner prior to a session for detailed precautions on that particular case.

Cervical Spine Problems

The spinal column is a protective shield surrounding the central nervous system, the main telecommunications network controlling all of the body's functions. The most threatening cervical spine problems occur when there is instability between the vertebrae of the spinal column.

Within the area of the cervical spine, the first seven vertebrae beginning at the base of the skull, there are two sets of arteries that operate as the main suppliers of blood and oxygen to the brain. The vertebral arteries travel along the back of the neck and the carotid arteries travel up the front of the neck. Any harm to the vertebrae or to the vertebral arteries could inflict permanent damage to the central nervous system. Examples of cervical spine problems include cervical hernia, arthrosis, osteoporosis, and cancer.

Precaution: Avoid all Thai Yoga Massage postures that induce spinal movement, especially all inverted exercises. A good workout with palming and thumbing on the sen lines can be applied in this case. As we get older we are more prone to cervical spine problems, so take care with older patients.

Constipation

Constipation is a bowel disorder that causes congestion of the colon and unusually difficult or infrequent bowel movements. A clockwise massage to the abdomen is good for stimulating bowel movements.

Precaution: Avoid the abdomen in case of acute stomachache.

Diarrhea

Diarrhea is a bowel disorder that causes abnormally frequent and watery bowel movements. A good massage on the back is recommended, as recipients with diarrhea may have a sore back.

Precaution: Do not work on the abdomen.

Dislocation

Dislocation is an abnormal placement of one bone in relationship to its articulation. A dislocation is usually brought on by an abrupt movement or by overextending or overstretching.

Precaution: Do not work on an area of dislocation. Do not overstretch an area of previous dislocation, as this could cause a relapse.

Fracture

Fracture is a break or crack in bone or cartilage. Certain conditions, such as osteoporosis and invasive cancer, make the bones fragile and easier to break.

Precaution: Do not work on or move a fractured bone, as this could cause a displacement of the broken pieces, thereby damaging surrounding tissue and delaying the healing process.

Hemophilia

Hemophilia is a rare disease in which blood is slow to clot. The disease affects men almost exclusively.

Precaution: Never work on clients with hemophilia. Massaging a person with this disease could generate external or internal bleeding. The consequence of either of these occurrences could be very dangerous to the individual.

Hernia

A hernia is a protrusion of an organ or other bodily structure through the wall that normally contains it. The most common hernias are spinal disc hernia and abdominal wall hernia.

Precaution: In the case of spinal disc hernia avoid all postures that flex or extend the spine, such as Cobra, Side Arc, and Locust. In the case of abdominal-wall hernia, avoid any flexion or extension of the abdomen or hip.

High Blood Pressure

A normal blood pressure reading for an adult is approximately 120 systolic/80 diastolic. Elevated blood pressure is a major risk factor for heart attack and stroke. This disease damages the arteries.

Precaution: Do not perform inverted postures, such as the Plough, Shoulderstands, and so forth. Never work on someone whose blood pressure is not under control unless you exclusively provide a gentle, calming massage along the sen lines.

Menstruation

Thai Yoga Massage can be helpful in relieving cramps during menstruation.

Precaution: Do not perform inverted postures during menstruation, avoid pressure on the lower abdomen during abdominal massage, and do not work on the marmas (pressure points).

Open Wounds and Cuts

Open wounds and cuts include all abnormal openings of the skin.

Precaution: Make sure all wounds are properly covered before beginning a session. Do not stretch the area around the wound, as this may prevent healing or cause a reopening of the wound.

Osteoporosis

Osteoporosis is a condition in which old bone breaks down and is not properly replaced by new bone tissue. The individual's bones become porous, fragile, and more likely to break. Osteoporosis is often referred to as the "silent thief," as it can progress painlessly and remain undiagnosed until a fracture occurs. According to the Osteoporosis Society of Canada, one in four women and one in eight men over the age of fifty are prone to osteoporosis.

Precaution: Avoid brisk movements and applying too much direct pressure, as this may cause bone breaks or fractures. Be especially careful when working on the cervical spine and chest.

Phlebitis

Phlebitis, or deep-vein thrombosis, is a disease that causes obstruction in the veins.

Precaution: Never work on the area of phlebitis, as you may displace the clot to another area.

Pregnancy

During pregnancy a woman's progesterone level is higher than usual. Pregnancy causes a woman's ligaments to relax and become less rigid, and as a result it is easier to harm joints and muscles while stretching and massaging. A gentle form of Thai Yoga Massage can help reduce cramps and labor pains in the lower back and legs.

Precaution: Be careful not to overstretch and do not apply pressure to the uterus. Do not work on the marmas (pressure points), and do not apply any inverted postures. From the second trimester on, a pregnant woman should not lie flat on her back for too long. The uterus and the baby are heavy in the abdomen and will compress the vena cava, the main vein at the back of the abdomen, decreasing the return of blood to the heart and thereby decreasing the woman's blood pressure. A decrease in blood pressure will reduce the amount of blood and oxygen going to the baby. Most pregnant women instinctively shift their bodies to the side; lying on the left side provides the most effective circulation to the uterus. This position will reduce the compression on the vena cava.

Rheumatoid Arthritis

Rheumatoid arthritis is an inflammation of the joints that endangers the stability of the bone. The inflammation causes joint damage, deformities of the joint articulations, and deterioration of the synovial bursae (joint capsules) and ligaments. If the practitioner is not careful he could dislocate a recipient's joint and bruise or tear the arteries or nerves. The damage to the arteries could obstruct the circulation of blood, and the damage to the nerves may result in paralysis.

When rheumatoid arthritis modifies the spine, the relationship between the vertebrae can be shifted. This may obstruct the spinal canal and squeeze the spinal cord, which can cause injury (especially in the cervical area).

Precaution: Never work on clients with rheumatoid arthritis unless you have a doctor's approval.

Skin Disease

Skin disease includes all abnormal skin conditions. Noncontagious skin diseases include acne, eczema, and skin allergies. Contagious skin diseases include athlete's foot and chicken pox.

Precaution: Avoid working on the infected area, except in cases such as athlete's foot, in which you can work through a pair of socks.

Surgery

Precaution: Do not perform Thai Yoga Massage on an area that has been operated on for at least one to three months, depending on the nature of the surgery. Massage can obstruct the healing process and cause sutures to burst.

Varicose Vein

A varicose vein is a vein that is abnormally dilated and has lost some ability to efficiently circulate blood back to the heart. A varicose vein can develop into phlebitis.

Precaution: Do not apply direct pressure to varicose veins; massaging surrounding tissues can improve local circulation.

—ന—

The concepts outlined in part 1 will guide you in giving a Thai Yoga Massage session with confidence, grace, and a still mind. With this introduction to theoretical and movement foundations, let's move on to learning the postures and flowing transitions of a Thai Yoga Massage session.

PART TWO

❖

The Practice

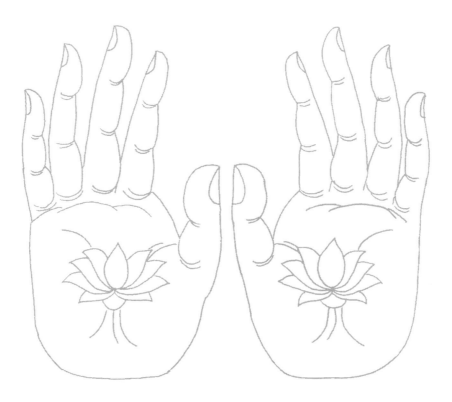

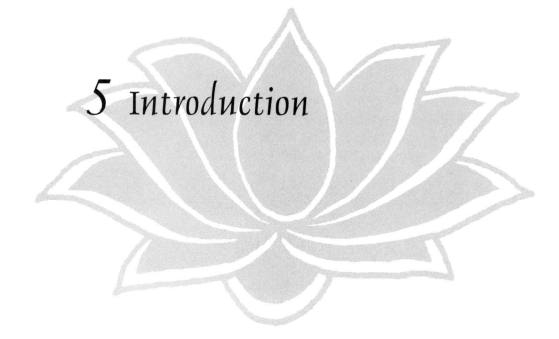

5 Introduction

Welcome to the practice section of this book. The following chapters will take you through a basic Thai Yoga Massage session. Each massage posture is clearly demonstrated, and instructions are provided for full and safe execution. Benefits, precautions, and adaptations for the recipient's ease are also indicated.

The chapters and postures are organized in accordance with the structure of a full-body Thai Yoga Massage and are presented according to two levels of massage: basic and extended. A basic session lasts approximately 1.5 hours and includes all poses in the chapter, except those beginning with a †. For an extended session of approximately 2.5 hours, include the postures indicated by the symbol †.

The session begins with the sitting postures and then moves on to double- and single-foot exercises, sen work on the legs, and single-leg exercises. These are followed by the side-lying postures, back-position postures, and double-leg exercises. The session finishes with restful massage of the abdomen, chest, arms, hands, and face.

It is useful to remember that every time you palm or thumb the feet, legs, abdomen, chest, arms, hands, back, and face, the sen energy lines are engaged. Many of the Thai Yoga Massage postures practiced here engage several energy lines at the same time. When the postures are correctly complemented with the techniques of palming and thumbing, a comprehensive bodywork strategy is achieved.

As noted in chapter 2, the rhythm and intensity of each pose can be linked to the three main Ayurvedic principles. For vata-dominant recipients the approach should be slow and gentle, for those of a pitta nature it should be nonvigorous and relaxing, and for kapha recipients the massage should be energetic and fiery.

As you practice these postures be mindful that you are maintaining one of the key stances: Diamond, Open Diamond, Kneeling Diamond, Cat 1, Cat 2, Cat 3, Warrior stance, Archer stance, or Tai Chi stance. When applying a technique, no matter how subtle, always bear in mind the rhythmic rocking dance methods of bamboo, forward, and whirlpool rock.

As a final note, remember to approach your work with ease. Be natural in your engagement, have fun, and always keep an inner smile! What a privilege it is to help others and to express the physical application of metta in motion.

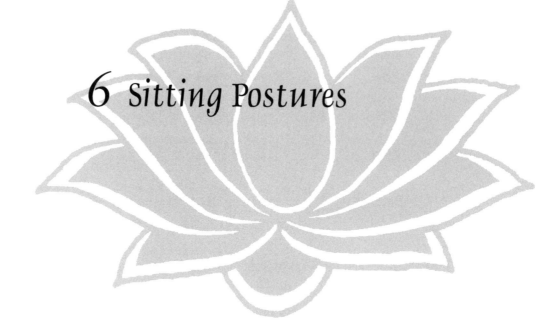

6 Sitting Postures

Because we in the West spend a lot of time sitting in chairs, often working in offices, our physical tension tends to accumulate most prominently in the upper body and neck area. As the saying goes, we carry the world's burdens on our shoulders, which can be a very heavy weight to bear. For that reason the Lotus Palm method of Thai Yoga Massage commences with the sitting position to address the shoulders first and to open up the upper body.

Figure 6.1 shows points of tension and vital points, or marmas, for relieving stress in the shoulders and scapula. Work along the indicated sen lines, listening with your hands. (The sen lines are shown in gray; see also pages 9–14 to see the sen lines in greater detail.) Rub, squeeze, and soothe any tension areas that you discover during the session. Do not use jerky movements, and especially avoid the infamous maneuver of cracking the neck.

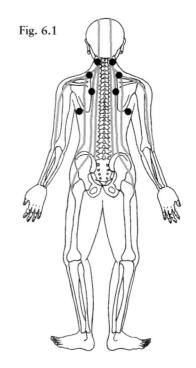

Fig. 6.1

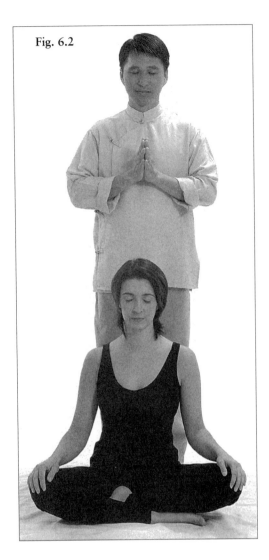

Fig. 6.2

Namaskar

Thai Yoga Massage begins with centering—focusing thought and spirit on the present moment and creating a sacred space. The practitioner stands behind the recipient, who is comfortably seated with legs crossed, or alternatively, with legs extended. The recipient's hands should be resting on her lap. The practitioner joins his palms together in a prayer gesture. The eyes close softly (**fig. 6.2**).

The purpose of this centering is to adopt an attitude of mindfulness, allowing the practice of moment-to-moment awareness. Distractions and negative thoughts are dispelled. With mindfulness the practitioner invites connection with the recipient and with the spirit of Thai Yoga Massage. Closely related to the practice of mindfulness is the practice of metta, or loving-kindness. The entire massage is carried out with mindfulness and metta. These two elements distinguish Thai Yoga Massage as a deep, lovingly meditative, and spiritual experience.

Adaptation: If the recipient is uncomfortable sitting on the floor, you can invite her to sit on a pillow.

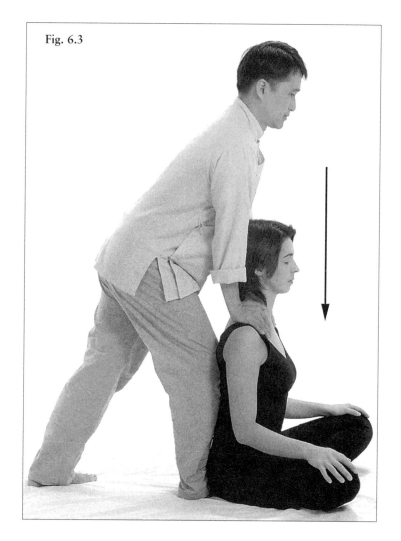

Fig. 6.3

Palming Shoulders

Using the Tai Chi stance, support the recipient's back with the lateral side of your right lower leg (tibialis anterior muscle). Note that the right heel is turned outward and the toes are turned slightly inward to make the fleshy part of the leg available to the recipient's back. Make sure the recipient is fully supported and her back is aligned.

Place your palms on top of the recipient's shoulders, keep your arms and back straight, and lean your bodyweight into the recipient's shoulders. The point of contact is on the trapez-ius muscle, not the clavicle. Use the forward rock to palm the shoulders. The direction of pressure is straight down (**fig. 6.3**).

Adaptation: For comfort, a pillow can be placed between your lower leg and recipient's back.

Benefits: Relieves tension in the trapezius muscles; increases shoulder and neck mobility.

Precaution: Avoid pressing on bones (the clavi-cle and the humerus), as this can be painful.

Recommended for: Vata and pitta

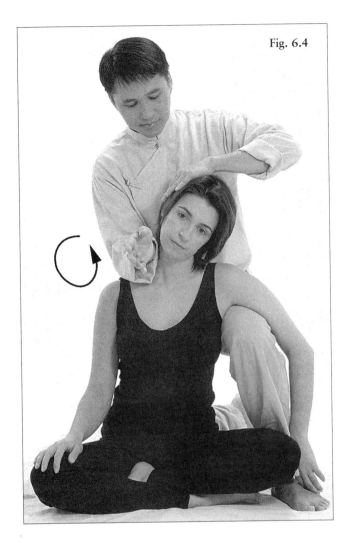

Fig. 6.4

Rolling Pin

From Tai Chi stance, move into the Kneeling Diamond stance while continuing to support the recipient's back with your hands. Then move into Warrior stance, maintaining contact with the recipient's back as you slide your left leg under the recipient's left arm.

Use your left hand to gently move the recipient's head toward her left shoulder, exposing and gently stretching the right trapezius muscle. Forward rock and roll your right forearm along the right upper trapezius muscle, from the base of the neck to the shoulder (**fig. 6.4**).

Move on to Cow Face 1.

Adaptation: For comfort, a pillow can be placed between your thigh and the recipient's back. This will help provide a comfortable separation between your bodies.

Benefits: Relieves tension in the trapezius muscles and relaxes the shoulders.

Precaution: Avoid rolling on bones (the clavicle or humerus).

Recommended for: Vata and pitta

Cow Face 1

Remaining in Warrior stance, use your right hand to grasp under the recipient's right elbow and your left hand to hold the recipient's hand. Lift and rotate the upper arm to warm up the shoulder (**fig. 6.5**).

Bring the recipient's elbow above the head, allowing the hand to fall behind the recipient's head. With both hands, gradually pull the elbow toward the center of your torso to stretch the triceps muscles (**fig. 6.6**). Fix the recipient's elbow to your torso with your left hand. Use your right hand to squeeze the triceps muscles, moving from the elbow down to the underarm (**fig. 6.7**). Release slowly, guiding the recipient's arm back to her lap.

If the recipient is quite flexible in Cow Face 1, the Water Pump and Cow Face 2 are good continuations. If the recipient is not so flexible through the shoulder and upper arm, repeat Rolling Pin and Cow Face 1 on the other side before moving on to Neck Massage. Remember that you must reverse your stance to work these postures on the opposite side.

Benefits: Mobilizes the scapula and shoulders; extends and relaxes the triceps.

Common mistake: The practitioner has the wrong knee raised in Warrior stance. Be sure that the raised knee supports the side opposite to the arm being worked. This will prevent the recipient from falling to the side.

Precaution: Be careful not to hyperextend the back by overstretching the arms. Avoid squeezing the armpit, which will aggravate the lymph nodes (and possibly tickle the recipient). Be careful not to pinch the recipient's skin with your fingernails.

Reccommended for: Vata and Pitta

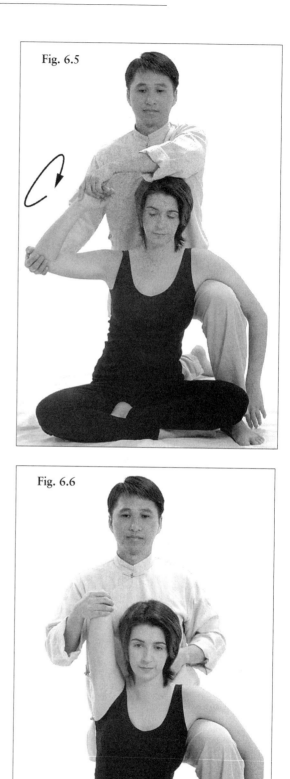

Fig. 6.5

Fig. 6.6

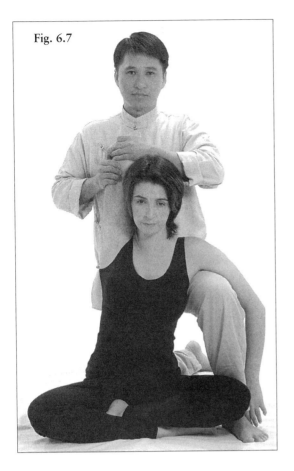

Fig. 6.7

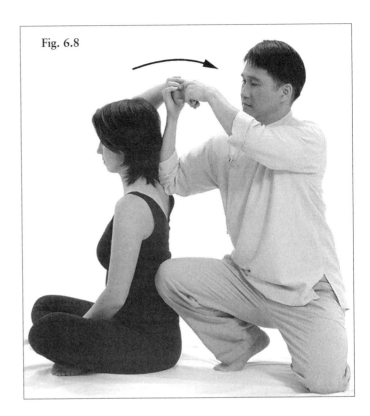

Fig. 6.8

✝ Water Pump

The Water Pump works the area between the scapula and the spine, which I affectionately refer to as the "ohh . . . this is great!" area. This posture is a stronger version of Cow Face 1.

Keeping the recipient's right arm elevated, move into Archer stance, your right knee supporting the left side of the recipient's back. Place your right elbow on the recipient's right trapezius muscle, near the neck. Use your right hand to grasp the recipient's right wrist. Hold the recipient's hand with your left hand.

Elbow the area between the scapula and the spine while pulling the recipient's arm toward you, as if pumping water (**fig. 6.8**). Elbow the

area from the top to the bottom of the scapula.

Move on to Cow Face 2.

Adaptation: A pillow will help to soften the feel of the knee against the back.

Benefits: Provides traction to the humerus, stretching the triceps muscles; works the muscles beside the scapula.

Precaution: This posture provides a deep stretch and should be used only if Cow Face 1 is met with no significant resistance. Take care not to elbow the spine.

Recommended for: Kapha

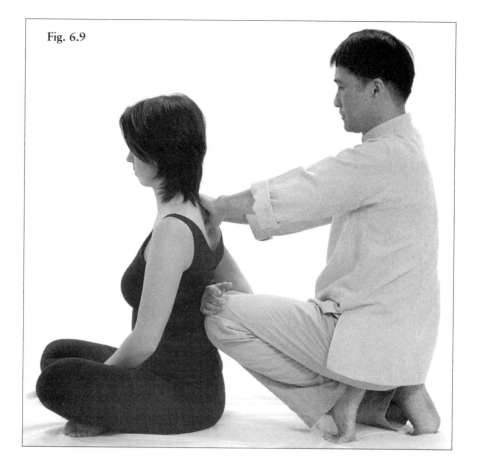

Fig. 6.9

† Cow Face 2

Alternate the Archer stance by moving onto your other knee. Place the recipient's arm behind her back in an "FBI" lock. This is accomplished by bringing the raised arm around behind the recipient's back and fixing the hand against the lower back with your left knee.

Grasp the right shoulder with the right hand and press behind the scapula with your left thumb (**fig. 6.9**). (At this point the recipient will usually make exclamations to the effect of "ohh . . . this is great!") Gradually move from the top to the bottom of the scapula.

Repeat all postures from Rolling Pin through Cow Face 2 on the opposite side.

Benefits: Provides deep massage of the subscapularis and rhomboid muscles, common areas for stress-related tension; increases range of motion of shoulders and arms.

Recommended for: Vata, pitta, and kapha

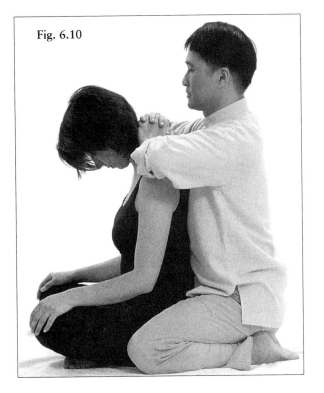

Fig. 6.10

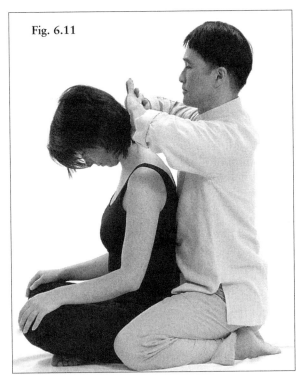

Fig. 6.11

Neck Massage

Move into Open Diamond stance. Straddle the recipient's body, allowing the recipient to be fully supported.

Push the recipient's head slightly forward to expose and elongate the neck. Interlace your fingers and massage the neck by gently squeezing together the heels of the palms (**fig. 6.10**).

Keeping your hands in the same interlaced position, forward rock and use your thumbs to massage the neck muscles along the cervical spine (**fig. 6.11**). Work these muscles as if you were picking up a cat by its neck.

Move on to Jade Pillow if you are performing an extended massage; if not move on to the Shampoo posture.

Adaptation: For comfort a pillow can be placed between your body and the recipient's. This will provide a respectful separation between bodies, and may be important for recipient's with a known history of sexual abuse.

Benefits: Tones the cervical and brachial plexus muscles, where the nerve roots to the neck, upper extremities, and upper torso are located; relieves tension in the neck, shoulders, and upper back; relieves headaches and nausea.

Precaution: Take care not to squeeze the sides of the neck. Compressing the sternocleidomastoid muscle in this way can be very uncomfortable. Be careful not to squeeze the cervical spine.

Recommended for: Vata and pitta

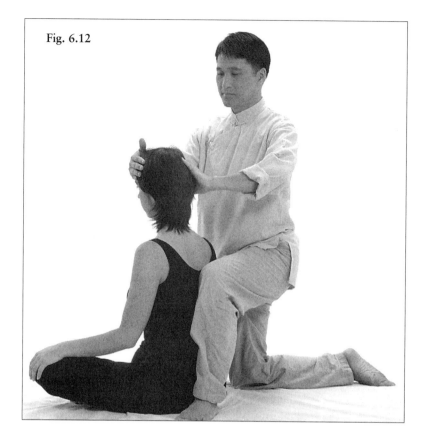

Fig. 6.12

✝ Jade Pillow

From the Open Diamond stance, move to the right side of the recipient and into the Warrior stance, your left knee raised. Support the recipient's back with the medial side of your left lower leg. Your torso and the recipient's torso are perpendicular.

Support the recipient's forehead with your right hand. Using the left hand, apply moderate thumb pressure along the base of the skull (**fig. 6.12**).

In one fluid motion, slide to the left side of the recipient, raising your right knee. (This will take practice!) Repeat the Jade Pillow massage on other side, then move on to the Shampoo posture.

Benefits: Stimulates the occipital nerves at the base of the skull, which relaxes the skull and forehead; massages arteries and lymph nodes, providing circulation throughout the head. This massage is good for healing headaches and clearing congestion or heaviness in the head.

Precaution: Be careful not to apply too much pressure. Avoid pressure on the carotid artery, located behind the ear.

Recommended for: Vata, pitta, and kapha

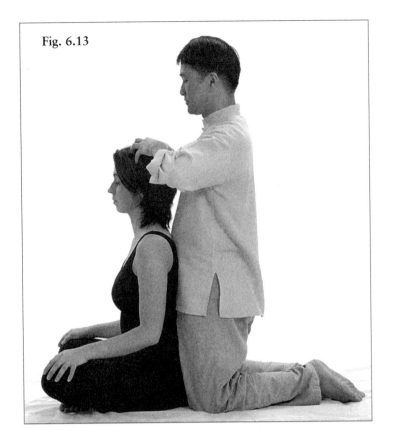

Fig. 6.13

Shampoo

Move into the Kneeling Diamond stance.

Support the recipient with your torso and massage the scalp with your fingertips, as if shampooing her hair (**fig. 6.13**).

Adaptation: For comfort, a pillow can be placed between your body and the recipient's.

Benefits: Stimulates the scalp and roots of the hair; strengthens hair and releases tension around the head.

Recommended for: Vata, pitta, and kapha

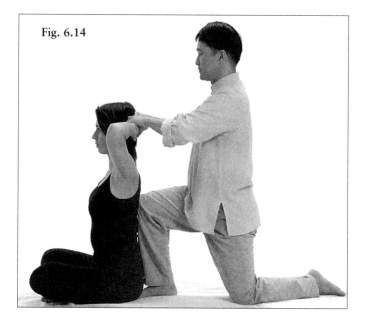

Fig. 6.14

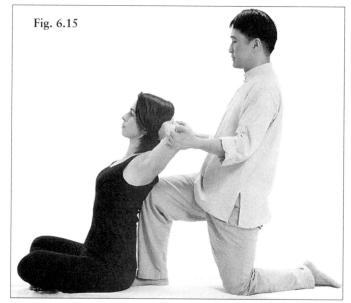

Fig. 6.15

Double Pec Stretch

Grasp the recipient's arms by the elbows; raise them up and interlace the fingers behind the head. Support the recipient's head with your hands and move into the Warrior stance, right knee raised (**fig. 6.14**). Support the recipient's spine with the right lower leg.

Grasp the elbows from below and direct your recipient to inhale. Direct her to exhale as you gradually pull back so her back bends over your knee (**fig. 6.15**). Stay in this position for two breaths, then slowly assist her back to the starting seated posture. Unclasp the recipient's hands,

gently guiding the arms back to her lap. Move on to Rowboat, or to Prayer Pose if you are performing a basic Thai Yoga Massage.

Adaptation: For comfort, a pillow can be placed between your leg and the recipient's back.

Benefits: Stretches the thoracic muscles, relieving chest congestion and tension; increases mobility of the shoulder and scapula; relieves tension in the pectoral and triceps muscles.

Recommended for: Kapha

† Rowboat

From Warrior stance move into Kneeling Diamond stance. Grasp the recipient's elbows and allow the hands to fall beside the hips. Support the recipient's shoulders with your hands.

Cross your legs behind you, roll back, and sit down in a cross-legged position (**fig. 6.16**).

Place your feet on the recipient's upper back, with your toes on the scapula. Grasp the recipient's wrists and gently lift and spread the arms outward, as if you are conducting an orchestra (**fig. 6.17**). Bend your legs at the knees, allowing the recipient to fall into an upper-back backbend (**fig. 6.18**).

Straighten your legs to gently push the recipient upright.

Repeat twice, moving your feet down the back about one inch at a time.

Benefits: Helps relax the back after sitting; strengthens the back by supporting the recipient in a properly upright posture.

Precaution: Be careful not to pull the arms too much, as this can cause discomfort to the shoulder and pectoral muscles.

Recommended for: Kapha, and for vata if performed gently

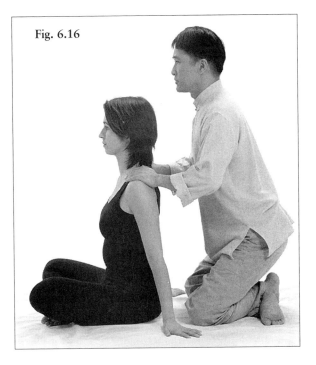

Fig. 6.16

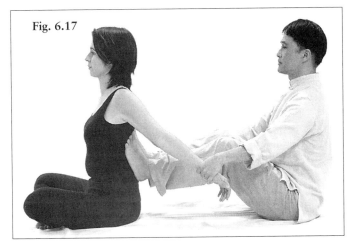

Fig. 6.17

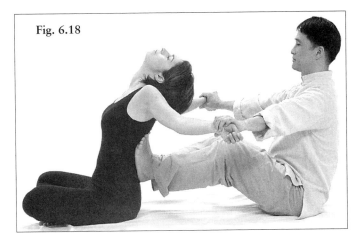

Fig. 6.18

Prayer Pose (Palming on Back)

A special transition is needed to move out of Rowboat pose in preparation for Prayer Pose. While maintaining a hold on the wrists, move your feet off the recipient's back and cross the legs in front of you, as if preparing for seated meditation (**fig. 6.19**). Roll up onto your knees and into Warrior stance, right leg raised, while simultaneously sliding your hands up the recipient's arms to the elbows (**fig. 6.20**).

Using the momentum from rolling up, swing the recipient forward so she bends at the waist, arms extended (**fig. 6.21**). This transition should be done in one fluid motion. Practice makes progress!

If you are coming into Prayer Pose from the Double Pec Stretch, gently bend the recipient forward at the waist, arms extended forward (**fig. 6.21**).

Palm up and down the muscles alongside the recipient's spine by forward rocking (**fig. 6.22**).

Adaptation: If the recipient is stiff or uncomfortable in this cross-legged position, she may extend her legs forward before bending forward. Place a cushion or pillow between the legs and the abdomen of a less flexible recipient.

Benefits: Relaxes and relieves back tension; counters the stretch of the Rowboat pose.

Recommended for: Vata

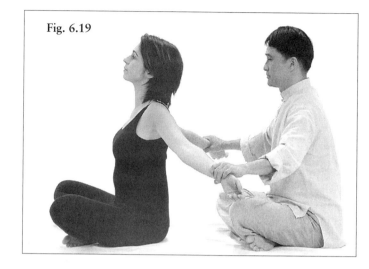

Fig. 6.19

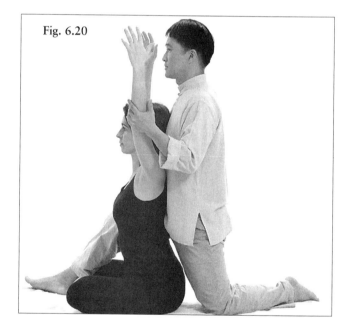

Fig. 6.20

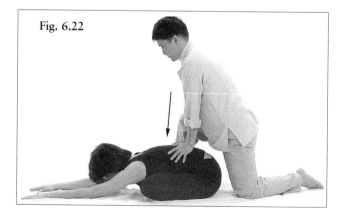

Fig. 6.22

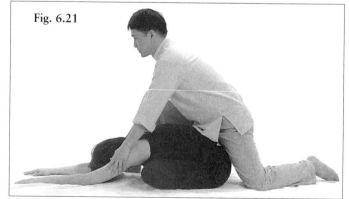

Fig. 6.21

Chopping

Remain in the Warrior stance with the recipient in Prayer Pose.

Press palms together and chop into the recipient's back, making a "clapping" sound (**fig. 6.23**).

Chopping is tricky, as your hands and fingers can easily slide out of place. Find the balance between soft and hard pressure in your hands. In the beginning, your hands might not stay together and the sound may be weak and unimpressive. Do it a few hundred times and you will get it for sure!

Benefits: Releases and disperses tension in the back.

Recommended for: Vata

Transitional Flow

With the recipient in the Prayer Pose and you in the Warrior stance, place both of your hands on the recipient's shoulders and pull her up into the sitting position. Drop into the Kneeling Diamond stance and knee-walk away from the recipient, supporting her neck and upper back. Gently lower her into the supine position as you move into the Diamond stance. Once the recipient is rested in the supine position, prepare for the foot exercises by walking toward her feet and sitting in the Cat 1 stance.

This concludes the sitting postures. We're now ready to move on to the double- and single-foot exercises.

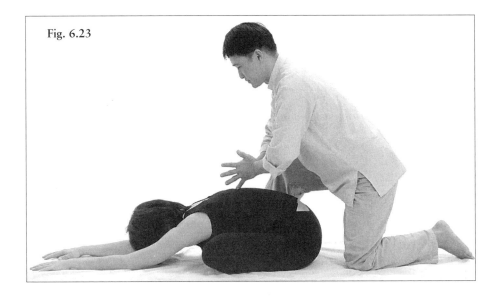

Fig. 6.23

7 Double- and Single-Foot Postures

In the science of reflexology, the various zones of the foot represent different regions of the body. On the sole of the foot, the tips of the toes represent the head, the instep corresponds to the internal organs, and the heel relates to the pelvic area, to name a few of the correspondences in reflexology. When massage therapists work on the feet they are actually influencing the whole body. For example, when we rotate the ankle we are also rocking the spine; by working on the instep we stimulate the digestive track. The reflex points on the feet are shown in figure 7.1. Massaging the reflex points on the feet further opens the body in preparation for the rest of the Thai massage session.

The first five movements in this part of the session work both feet simultaneously. Once you reach the Foot and Ankle Rotation, perform all the remaining movements on one foot and then switch to the other foot.

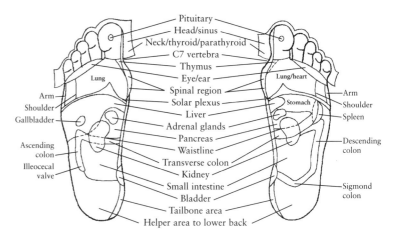

Fig. 7.1

72

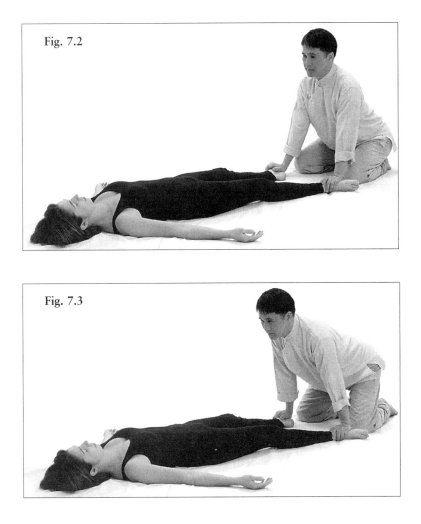

Fig. 7.2

Fig. 7.3

Palming Instep

In the Cat 1 stance, spread the recipient's feet shoulder-width apart. Place your hands on the recipient's insteps, keeping back and arms straight (**fig. 7.2**).

Palm the recipient's insteps by forward rocking in the Cat 3 stance, leaning in with your bodyweight to stretch and open the foot (**fig. 7.3**). Begin close to the heel and gradually palm toward the ball of the foot.

Repeat three times.

Benefits: Stretches and opens up the feet and the soleus muscles; tones the stomach, bladder, pancreas, and kidneys by working the correspon-

ding reflexology points on the feet; alleviates fatigue in the feet and legs.

Precaution: In the case of knee problems, proceed gently.

Common mistakes: The practitioner's back is curved and his head is down while rocking toward the recipient. It is important to keep your head up and your back straight, and to watch the recipient's face for signs of discomfort. Another problem is placing the recipient's feet too far apart. Spreading the feet farther than shoulder-width apart will place undue strain on the knees.

Recommended for: Vata, pitta, and kapha

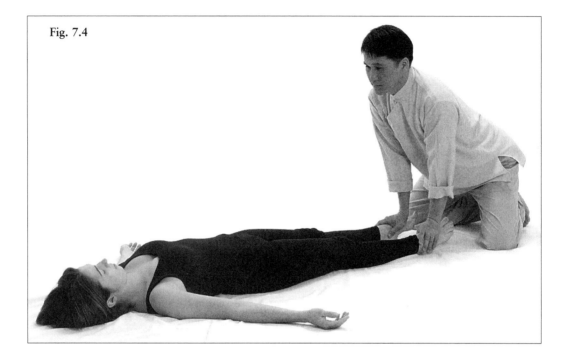

Fig. 7.4

† Palming Feet (Plantarflexion)

In the Cat 1 stance, adjust the recipient's feet upright and push on the heels so that the toes extend pointing toward you. Place your hands on the dorsal side of the feet, close to the ankles.

Forward rock in the Cat 3 stance, leaning in with your bodyweight (**fig. 7.4**).

Repeat three times.

Benefits: Flexes and activates the gastrocnemius muscles; provides traction to the tibia and femur, stretching the tibialis anterior muscles; alleviates fatigue in the feet and legs; alleviates arthrosis, stiff ankles, knee pain, and numbness in the lower extremities.

Recommended for: Vata, pitta, and kapha

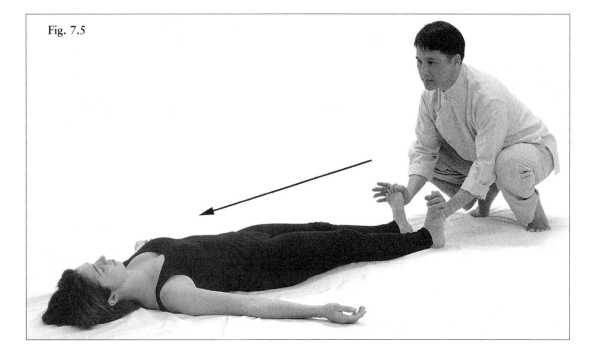

Fig. 7.5

† Pushing Ball of Foot (Dorsiflexion)

From a squatting position, adjust the recipient's feet so the toes point upright.

Grasp the balls of the recipient's feet. Fix your elbows on the inside of your knees for leverage. Flex the ankles by leaning into the balls of the feet (**fig. 7.5**). Hold for ten seconds and then gently release.

Benefits: Stretches the Achilles tendon and the entire lower back; alleviates fatigue in the feet and legs; alleviates arthritis, stiff ankles, lower back ache, and sciatica.

Recommended for: Vata and pitta

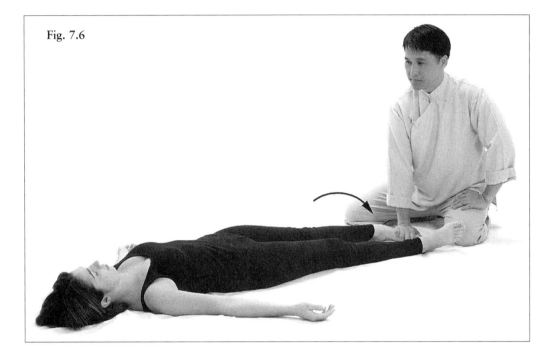

Fig. 7.6

Footfold

Sit in Open Diamond stance and spread the recipient's feet shoulder-width apart. Use your hands to alternately fold the recipient's feet gently inward, gradually pushing one and then the other sole flat onto the mat (**fig. 7.6**). Repeat this movement three times with each foot.

Benefits: Stretches the peroneus muscles; stimulates digestion by working on corresponding reflexology points; alleviates fatigue in the feet and legs; alleviates arthrosis and stiff ankles.

Precaution: In the case of knee problems, proceed gently. Also note that recipients with stiff ankles won't have the flexibility to move their feet all the way down to the mat.

Recommended for: Vata, pitta, and kapha

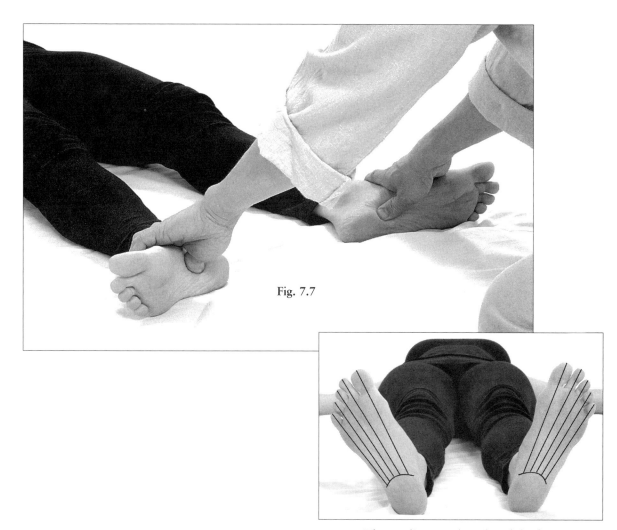

Fig. 7.7

The sen lines on the soles of the feet.

Thumbing Sen on Sole

Like a sun spreading its rays, the energy lines on the sole of the foot extend from the heel to the tip of each toe.

In Cat 1 stance with your arms and back straight, place your thumbs on the recipient's soles (**fig. 7.7**). Forward rock with your thumbs to tonify each energy line on the feet, beginning with the line running to the big toe and ending with the line running to the small toe. Don't be surprised if you hear snoring at this point in the massage!

Benefits: Stimulates the intrinsic muscles and nerves of the plantar region of the foot; helps balance the major organs, glands, and body systems according to reflexology principles; reduces insomnia.

Precaution: Avoid strong pressure on these energy lines if the recipient is pregnant.

Recommended for: Vata, pitta, and kapha

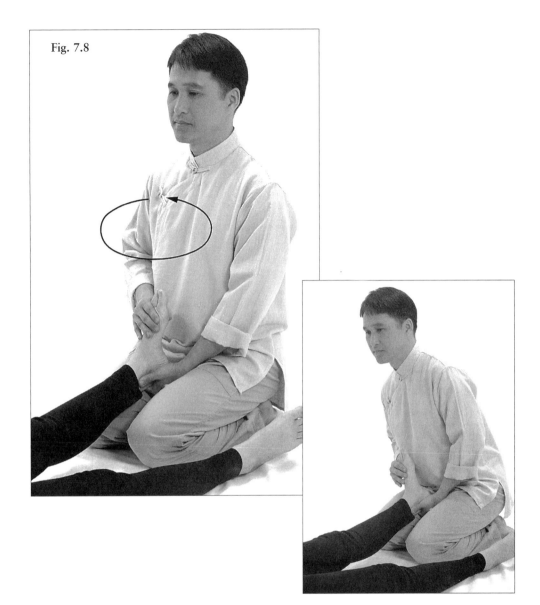

Fig. 7.8

Foot and Ankle Rotation

Sit in Diamond stance with the recipient's leg resting between your thighs and the bottom of her foot close to your belly. Cup the heel with one hand and use your other hand to hold the ball joints.

Using the whirlpool rock, rotate the ankle in a full circle (**fig. 7.8**). Repeat three times on each side.

Benefits: Mobilizes joints between the tarsal and metatarsal bones of the foot, loosening up the ligaments in this (usually very tight) area; limbers up the ankle and foot; relaxes the spinal column.

Common mistake: Recipient's foot is too far away from the practitioner's body.

Recommended for: Vata and pitta

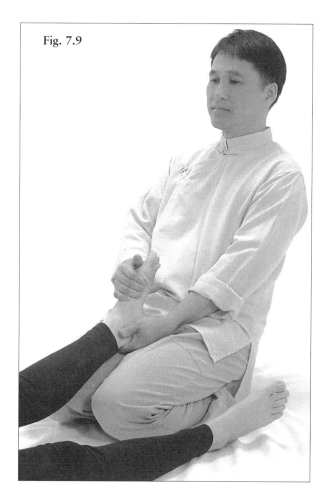

Fig. 7.9

† Foot Spinal Twist

Sit in Diamond stance with recipient's leg on top of your thighs and her foot close to your belly. Cup the heel with one hand and use the other hand to hold the foot across the top of the toes.

Fall back, allowing the foot to twist in your hand (**fig. 7.9**). Use your full bodyweight when leaning back to maximize the stretch. Repeat on the opposite side of the same foot.

Benefits: Gives a strong inversion stretch to the tibialis anterior and an eversion stretch to the peroneus longus and brevis muscles; relieves arthrosis, stiff ankle, spinal inflexibility, and insomnia.

Common mistake: Recipient's foot is not resting on the practitioner's lap.

Recommended for: Vata and pitta

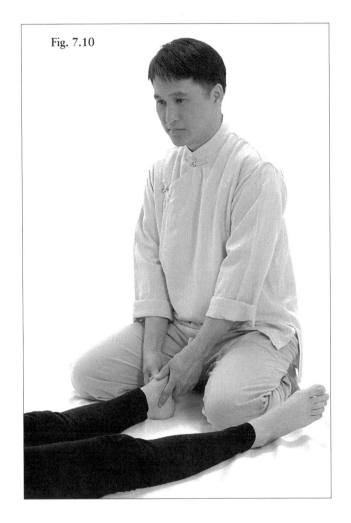

Fig. 7.10

Thumbing Sen on Dorsal

Place the recipient's foot on the mat between your knees.

In Open Diamond stance, forward rock with your bodyweight to thumb into energy lines on the dorsal side of the foot (**fig. 7.10**). Follow each line from the ankle to the toe, and give each toe a gentle squeeze.

Benefits: Massages the metatarsal interosseous spaces, where nerves and veins pass through.

Common mistake: Practitioner raises his shoulders due to improper distance from recipient's foot. Relax your shoulders!

Recommended for: Vata, pitta, and kapha

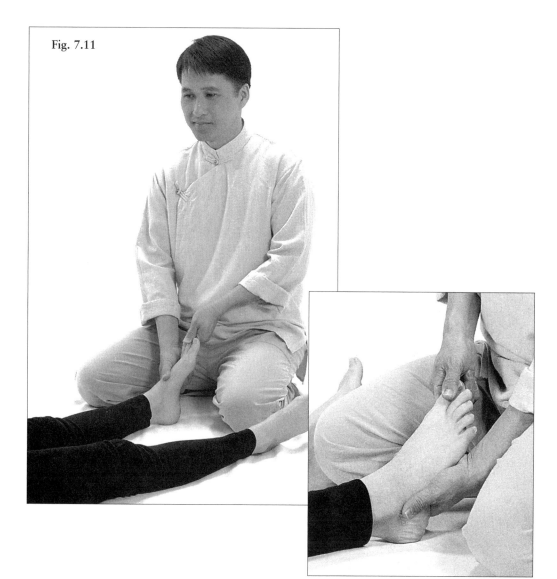

Fig. 7.11

✝ Toe Cracking

This is a favorite maneuver of Thai masseurs, but it isn't everyone's "cup of tea" so ask your recipient if she wants this part of the massage before proceeding.

Still in Open Diamond stance and with the recipient's foot on the mat between your knees, hold the sole of the foot with one hand. Use your other hand to firmly grasp each toe as you work.

Begin with the small toe. In a quick and confident move, pull the toe toward you to open the joint at the base of the toe (**fig. 7.11**). This move may release air bubbles trapped between joints and cause a "popping" effect.

Proceed with each toe.

Benefits: Relaxes the toes and clears lactic acid from the joints.

Precaution: If you don't hear the toes crack, don't pull harder!

Recommended for: Vata

Milk the Cow

Still in Open Diamond stance, place the recipient's foot on the mat between your knees. Moving from your hips, rock your bodyweight from side to side using the bamboo rock and using your hands to squeeze and soothe the foot (**figs. 7.12 and 7.13**).

Benefits: Provides a relaxing final touch to the foot exercises.

Recommended for: Vata, pitta, and kapha

Return to the Foot and Ankle Rotation and perform all the single-foot exercises on the other foot. To end the single-foot exercises, caress all parts of the recipient's foot and listen for "oohs" and "aahs."

❖

Transitional Flow

Move to the recipient's left side and take position in the Cat 1 stance.

This is the end of the foot exercises. We're ready to move on to the sen work on the legs and the single-leg postures.

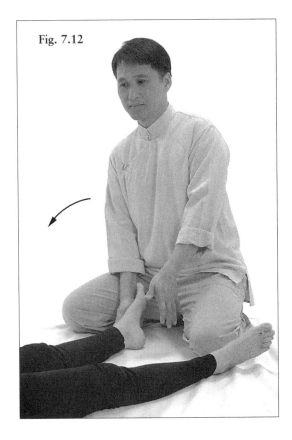

Fig. 7.12

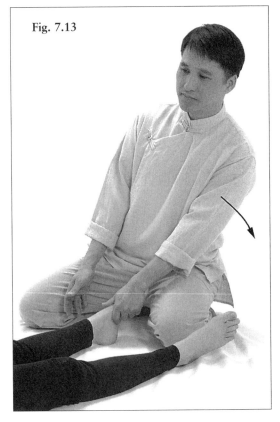

Fig. 7.13

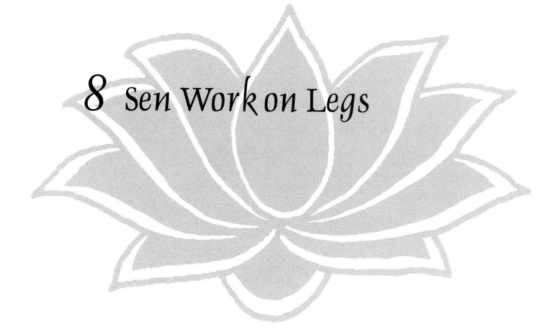

8 Sen Work on Legs

There are three sen lines that run along the medial side of the leg and three that run along the lateral side (**fig. 8.1**). In Thai Yoga Massage we use the technique of palming and thumbing to tonify these energy lines.

Thai Yoga Massage practitioners must be aware of their body mechanics, listen well with their hands, and watch the recipient's face for signs of discomfort. Generally speaking, the upper leg on either side of the thigh is more sensitive than the lower leg when applying palming and thumbing pressure. One can adjust to this difference by reducing the amount of pressure used on the upper leg. The amount of pressure a recipient can handle can be a little tricky to discern, and the need to respond to the recipient's comfort range demands your full attention.

Some of my students complain that sen work on the legs is the most boring part of the massage. My answer to that is that they should practice more meditation. In comparison to meditation, palming and thumbing are like aerobics.

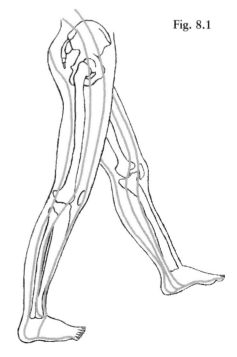

Fig. 8.1

When palming and thumbing the sen on the legs, first do the medial (inside) side of the leg farthest from you, and then the lateral (outside) side of the leg closest to you. Move to the recipient's other side and repeat.

Palming Sen

Sit in the Cat 1 stance alongside the recipient, aligning the midline of your torso with recipient's knee. Place one hand on the recipient's inside ankle and your second hand above the inside knee (**fig. 8.2**).

Gradually palm the leg using bamboo rocking, moving from ankle to knee and knee to upper thigh (**fig. 8.3 and 8.4**).

Benefits: Acts as an assistant pump to the heart, increasing the rate of blood flow without causing any strain to the heart. Removes waste materials through the venous and lymphatic systems.

Recommended for: Vata, pitta, and kapha

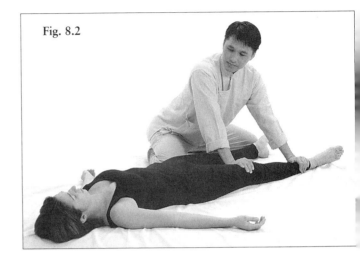

Fig. 8.2

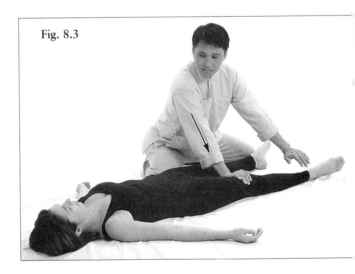

Fig. 8.3

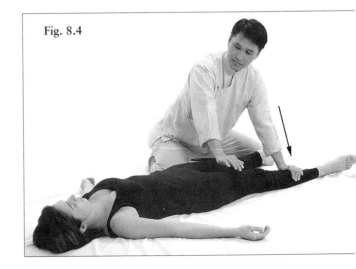

Fig. 8.4

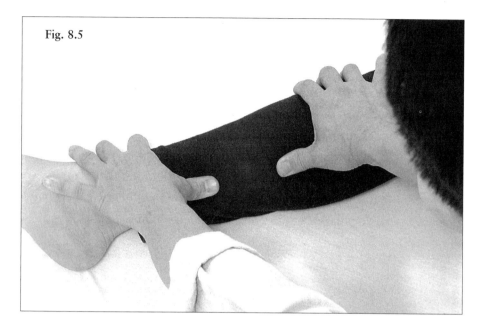

Fig. 8.5

Thumbing Sen

Sitting in the Cat 1 stance, you will continue the massage on the leg that was just palmed using the bamboo rocking technique. Use a thumb-chasing-thumb method to work along the sen of the lower leg (**fig. 8.5**).

Thumb the lower leg up and down between the ankle and the knee. Thumb the upper leg up and down between the knee and the upper thigh.

End with one more round of palming this leg, then move to the recipient's other side and perform palming and thumbing on that leg.

Benefits: Induces circulation along the principle arteries; alleviates numbness and fatigue in the legs.

Common mistake: The practitioner is not close enough to the recipient's leg and needs to reach too far forward.

Precaution: Avoid applying pressure to the knees; apply only light pressure on cellulite and varicose veins. Some varicose veins are very painful, and in this case pressure should be avoided entirely.

Recommended for: Vata, pitta, and kapha

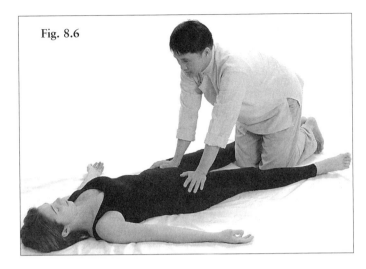

Fig. 8.6

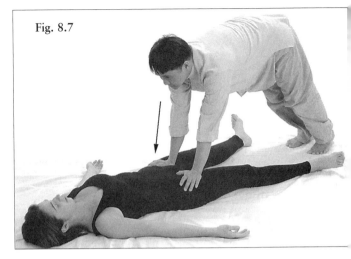

Fig. 8.7

† Blood Stop on Leg

Place the recipient's legs two feet apart and kneel in Cat 3 stance between her knees. Walk your palms up the leg to the area just below the groin. Apply gentle pressure to find the pulsation of the femoral arteries. Once you find it, move your hands down two inches (**fig. 8.6**).

Lift your tailbone and straighten your legs. This increases pressure on the recipient's upper thighs and stops the blood flow to the legs (**fig. 8.7**).

Hold for 60 seconds and release. The recipient should feel a warm tingling sensation moving down the thighs toward the toes.

Benefits: Clears the blood vessels and aids blood circulation.

Common mistake: The practitioner is straining to maintain an unstable stance. Come out of position if you feel unsteady or begin to tremble.

Precaution: Do not perform the Blood Stop on pregnant women, or on recipients with heart problems, varicose veins, or untreated high blood pressure. Avoid pressing on the inguinal lymph nodes beside the pelvic area. This area can be very irritable.

Recommended for: Kapha

❖

Transitional Flow

Drop into Cat 1 stance and move to the recipient's left side.

We're now ready to move on to the single-leg postures.

9 Single-Leg Postures

For the majority of my students the single-leg exercises are the most enjoyable and yet the most challenging aspect of performing a Thai Yoga Massage bodywork session. The focus on transitions here places great importance on the practitioner's tai-chi and body-centering skills.

The more graceful your dance through this section, the more beneficial the massage is for the recipient. Mastery of the transitions in this series will enable you to instill a feeling of confidence in the recipient, which thereby helps her to relax. She should feel as though she is drifting from one posture to another, like floating in water. If you begin to stumble and miss a step, the recipient may have trouble letting go.

I often ask my students to first practice the single-leg postures alone, without a recipient, a practice that I call shadow dancing. The result is a beautiful tai chi–like performance. As you practice these transitions be careful not to rush: wait until you have mastered one exercise before moving on to the next. I always advise my students to rehearse the series until the movements become fluid and natural. In my experience, if you can perform the single-leg exercises with ease you can go a long way in Thai Yoga Massage.

When performing the single-leg exercises, do all of the poses on one leg first and then walk around and work on the other side. For the sake of photographic clarity the images in this chapter sometimes switch from leg to leg. Don't be confused! Begin on one side of the body and perform the entire sequence of single-leg exercises there before switching to the other side.

Tree

Sitting in Diamond stance, hold the recipient's lower leg. Rotate the entire leg, warming up the hip joint (**fig. 9.1**).

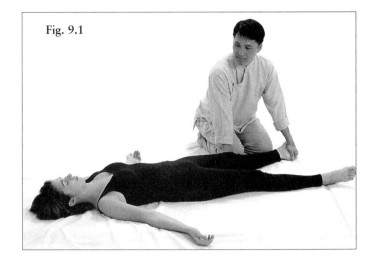

Fig. 9.1

Come into Warrior stance; make sure your stance is wide and stable. Lay the working leg down gently into the yoga Tree pose, bringing the sole of the recipient's foot to rest at the top of her inner thigh (**fig. 9.2**). Gently fix the knee to the mat with one hand; palm up and down the inner thigh with your other hand (**fig. 9.3**). You are often able to feel the tightness in the adductor muscles, the inside muscles of the leg.

For an extended Thai Yoga Massage session move on to High Heel posture. If you're performing a basic Thai Yoga Massage, stay in Warrior stance and move on to Angel Twist.

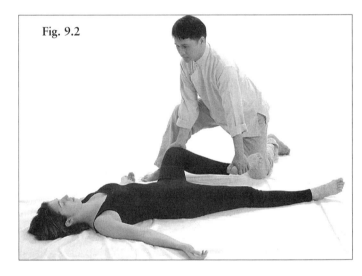

Fig. 9.2

Adaptation: Support the recipient's working knee with a pillow, if necessary, to relieve tension in the lower back.

Benefits: Stretches the adductor muscles and opens up the hip joint; increases mobility of the hip; compresses the abductor muscles to release tension in the outer leg.

Recommended for: Pitta

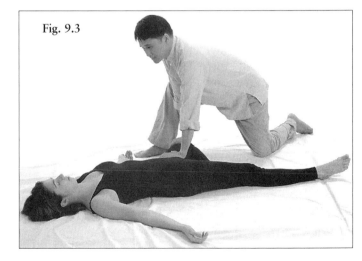

Fig. 9.3

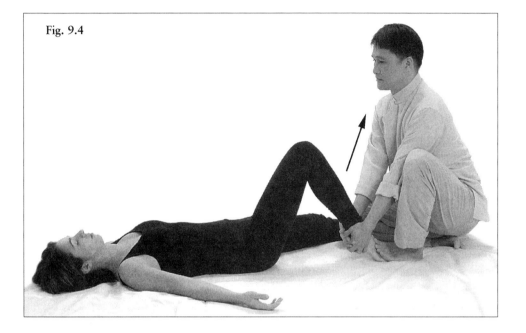

Fig. 9.4

✝ High Heel

From the Tree posture, lift the recipient's working knee so her foot is flat on the mat. Sit back on one heel and place your foot gently on top of the recipient's foot. Interlace your fingers and cup your hands under the recipient's heel.

Lift the recipient's heel by leaning back, giving a good heel stretch (**fig. 9.4**).

Benefits: Compresses the soleus muscle in the lower part of the calf; limbers up the ankle; relieves arthritis and foot fatigue.

Common mistake: The practitioner puts too much pressure on the recipient's foot.

Recommended for: Vata and kapha

Angel Twist

If you are coming to Angel Twist from the Tree posture, make sure to work on the same side as you were working in the Tree. You should perform all of the single-leg exercises on one side of the body before moving to the other side. The photographs here have switched to the recipient's right side for visual clarity only.

In the Warrior stance, push the recipient's knee toward the opposite thigh (**fig. 9.5**). Fix the knee with your closest hand and use your other hand to palm the iliotibial tract (**fig. 9.6**). Keep your arm straight as you palm and fall in with your bodyweight.

Move on to Side Kick, or to Knee to Forehead if you're performing a basic Thai Yoga Massage session.

Adaptation: Place a pillow between recipient's thighs to avoid discomfort in the knees and groin.

Benefits: Gently compresses and nourishes the intervertebral disks; releases the iliotibial tract; increases mobility and flexibility in the lower back; alleviates sciatica; releases tension on the upper thigh.

Recommended for: Vata and pitta

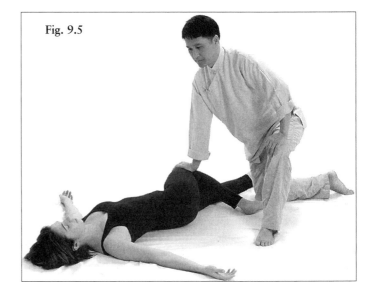

Fig. 9.5

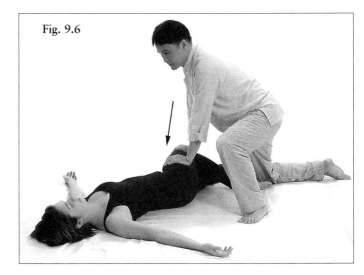

Fig. 9.6

✝ Side Kick

In the Warrior stance, straighten the recipient's leg (**fig. 9.7**). Rotate the entire leg, warming up the hip joint (**fig. 9.8**).

Gradually slide the leg out to the side at floor level until you feel resistance. Use your ankle to fix the recipient's ankle.

Place one hand on the recipient's knee and palm the inner thigh with your other hand (**fig. 9.9**). Martial artists love this movement because it helps them develop a more efficient side kick!

Benefits: Stretches adductor and hamstring muscles; improves mobility of hip joints; releases tension in the inner thigh (an area of the body that is often very tight).

Recommended for: Pitta and kapha

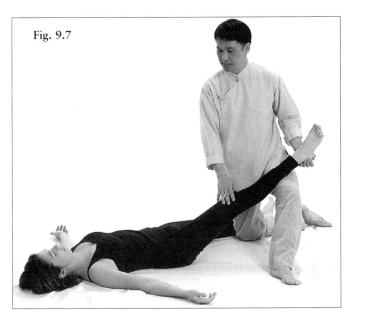

Fig. 9.7

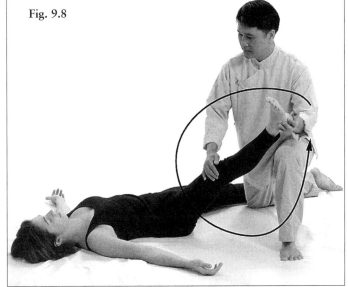

Fig. 9.8

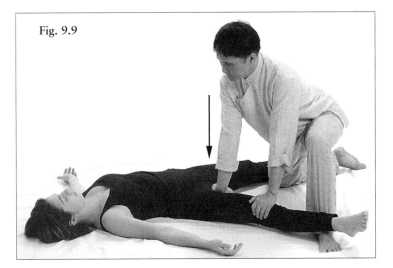

Fig. 9.9

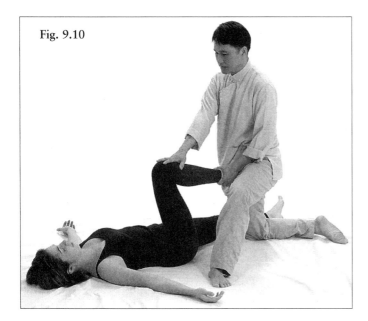

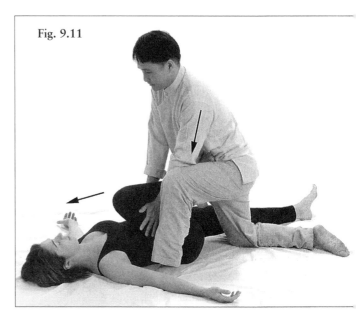

Knee to Forehead

In the Warrior stance, raise the recipient's leg and rest her foot on your pelvis, close to your hip joint (**fig. 9.10**).

With your palms on the recipient's hamstrings rock forward, guiding the knee to the forehead. Simultaneously palm up and down the hamstrings three times (**fig. 9.11**). The trajectory of the knee is headward while the force of your palming is in toward the belly and downward toward the floor.

Benefits: Stretches the knee and hip flexors; compresses and massages the hamstring muscles; improves mobility of hip; relieves gassy and bloated stomach.

Common mistake: Practitioner's bent knee exceeds his toes, causing an unsteady stance when rocking forward.

Precaution: Avoid this movement in cases of hernia, heart disease, and pregnancy.

Recommended for: Vata

Hurricane Kick

In the Warrior stance, "wag the tail," pivoting on your kneeling knee and sliding that lower leg inward approximately 40 degrees. Sit down and back while holding the recipient's leg in front of you (**fig. 9.12**).

Straighten your leg and place the blade of your foot behind the recipient's knee (**fig. 9.13**). Use your leg to bring the recipient's leg down to the mat, and hook the foot inside your knee (**fig. 9.14**).

Hold the recipient's ankles with your hands for support while you gently push the sole of your other foot into the hamstrings (**fig. 9.15**). Work your way down the length of the hamstrings.

Benefits: Compresses the knee flexors; kneads the muscles and releases tension in the upper leg.

Common mistake: In the early part of this movement be careful not to bring the recipient's foot down with you when you sit back, as this could break the flow of the movement.

Recommended for: Kapha, and for vata if done gently

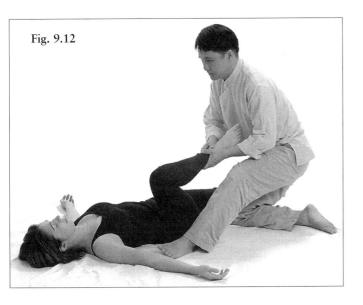

Fig. 9.12

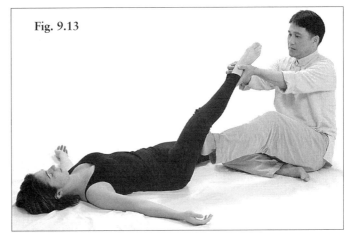

Fig. 9.13

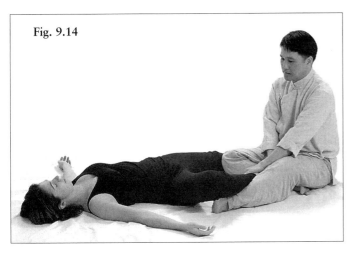

Fig. 9.14

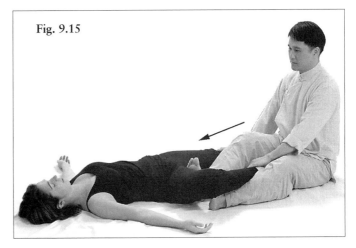

Fig. 9.15

Knee Stretch

From the Hurricane Kick, slide close to recipient's extended leg. Place the foot with which you palpated the hamstrings in Hurricane Kick over the recipient's free leg. Unhook the recipient's foot and place your instep under her knee (**fig. 9.16**).

Lift your working leg, bending the recipient's knee to a 90-degree angle.

Adjust your instep behind the knee; your toes are pointing out. Grasp the ankle and foot and let your bodyweight fall back to create a knee stretch (**fig. 9.17**).

Move on to Uranus for an extended Thai Yoga Massage session, or to Snake Creeps Down.

Adaptation: Wrap a towel around the recipient's foot to avoid pinching and discomfort.

Benefits: Opens the popliteal area behind the knee; creates space for the knee joint.

Common mistake: Not maintaining proper body alignment relative to the recipient's body. Be sure to lean straight back while pulling the recipient's leg so as not to rotate the knee. Take care not to pinch the ankle and heel.

Precaution: Proceed gently if the recipient has knee problems.

Recommended for: Vata and kapha

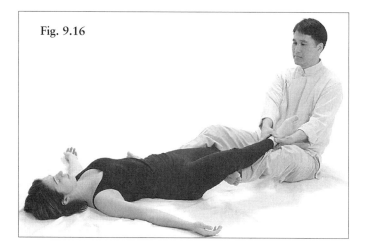

Fig. 9.16

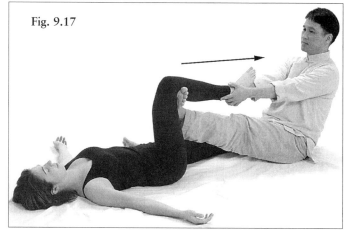

Fig. 9.17

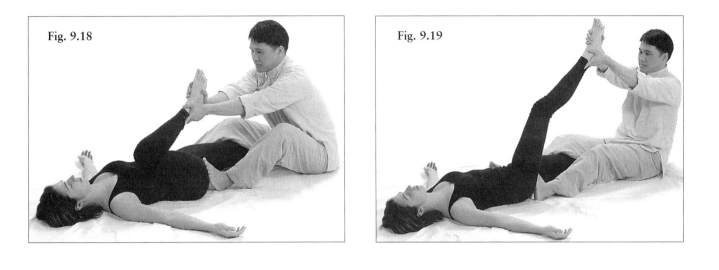

Fig. 9.18

Fig. 9.19

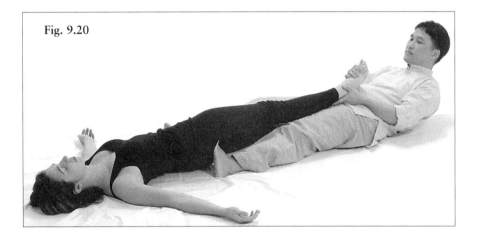

Fig. 9.20

⚕ Uranus

This posture is an advanced movement that requires steadiness, as a lack of control could cause a slip into the recipient's groin. From the Knee Stretch, continue to hold the recipient's ankle with your hands as you slide your foot down to the buttock. Gently push the recipient's knee toward her forehead and position the ball of your foot firmly on her sitz bone (**fig. 9.18**).

Pull the recipient's leg straight toward you while sliding your heel under the buttock, lifting the hip (**fig. 9.19**). Gently lean back and straighten the recipient's leg for a full hip-joint stretch (**fig. 9.20**). Your toes should be pressing upward just below the sitz bone.

Benefits: Stimulates and relieves tension in the sciatic nerves; relaxes the lower back; flexes the hips.

Common mistake: Your toes are too close to the anus. If your foot is not aligned under the sitz bone this movement will put great strain on your foot and toes.

Recommended for: Pitta and kapha

Snake Creeps Down

Again, in coming into this posture from Knee Stretch or Uranus make sure to continue working on the same side of the body.

Cross your legs and roll up into the Warrior stance, once again bending the knee of the recipient's working leg. While holding the ankle with both hands (**fig. 9.21**), rock forward into the Kneeling Diamond stance (**fig. 9.22**) and shift to the side of the recipient (**fig. 9.23**).

Fix one hand just above the recipient's knee and shift the other hand to cup the recipient's heel (**fig. 9.24**). Dorsiflex the foot by gradually straightening the arm that cups the recipient's heel.

Benefits: Works the intrinsic muscles of the foot and ankle, and the plantar flexor and hip extensor muscles; stretches the back of the legs and the lower back.

Common mistake: This stretch is effective only if the practitioner uses the area above the elbow for leverage. A tense shoulder reduces the effectiveness of the stretch.

Precaution: Avoid putting pressure on the recipient's knee. Your hand is on the thigh only for support.

Recommended for: Vata and kapha

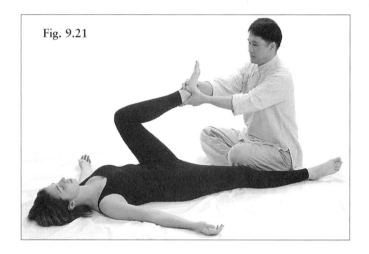

Fig. 9.21

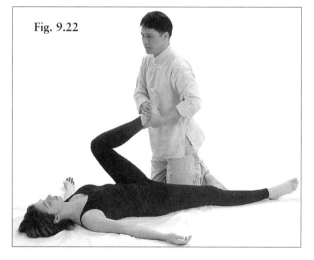

Fig. 9.22

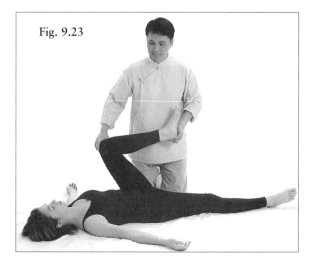

Fig. 9.23

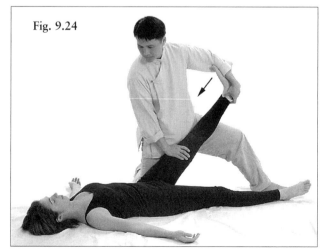

Fig. 9.24

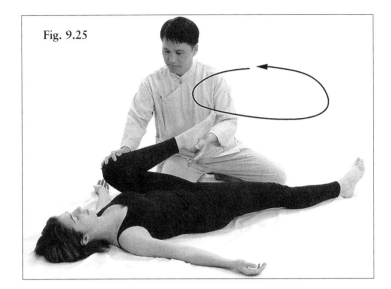

Fig. 9.25

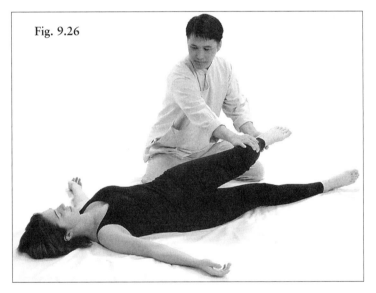

Fig. 9.26

Helicopter
(Knee and Hip Rotation)

With the hands still in place on the knee and the heel, sit down in Open Diamond stance and let the recipient's leg rest on your lap.

Use whirlpool rocking to rotate the recipient's knee and hip (**figs. 9.25 and 9.26**).

For an extended Thai Yoga Massage session, move on to the Diva Twist, which benefits recipients who are very flexible and not too heavy. If you're performing a basic Thai Yoga Massage,

perform all the Single-Leg Postures on the other side of the body.

Benefits: Mobilizes and limbers up the hip joint; relieves tension in the hip and leg; provides greater range of motion in the hips.

Common mistake: Practitioners do not rock with the whole body.

Recommended for: Vata, pitta, and kapha

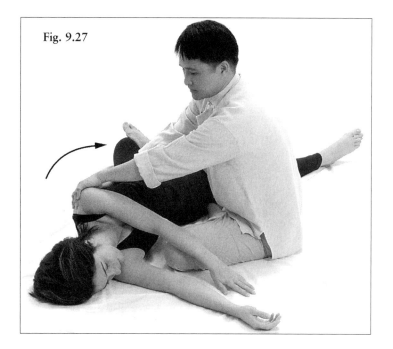

Fig. 9.27

⚕ Diva Twist

Lay the leg down gently into Tree posture. Walk around to the other side of the recipient's body.

Sit beside the recipient and drape your leg over hers, fixing your foot on top of the recipient's bent knee. Pull the recipient's shoulder toward you, giving her a gentle spinal twist (**fig. 9.27**).

If you've just completed the single-leg postures on the first side of the body, gently release the recipient back to supine and move to the recipient's other side.

Benefits: Rotates the thoracic spine, gently compressing the intervertebral disks; tractions the scapula; encourages mobility of the upper body; massages the paravertebral muscles.

Common mistake: Practitioner's bent knee presses into the ribs of the recipient. You can prevent this by placing a pillow between your knee and the recipient's ribs.

Precaution: Go easy as this twist can be painful, and it can be difficult for the practitioner to gauge his strength.

Recommended for: Vata, pitta, and kapha

❖

Transitional Flow

The basic Thai Yoga Massage session moves from the Helicopter (**see figures 9.25 and 9.26**) to the prone position in preparation for the back-position exercises. At the end of Helicopter ask the recipient to rest her arms above her head. With the momentum of the Whirlpool rock, swing her knee while you step into Warrior stance with your front foot over her outside leg. Gently swing the recipient onto her abdomen.

The transition for the extended session moves from the Diva Twist to the side-lying position. Simply release your working leg from the recipient's knee and gently roll her onto her side. The side-lying postures are included in an extended Thai Yoga Massage and introduce a more advanced level of practice.

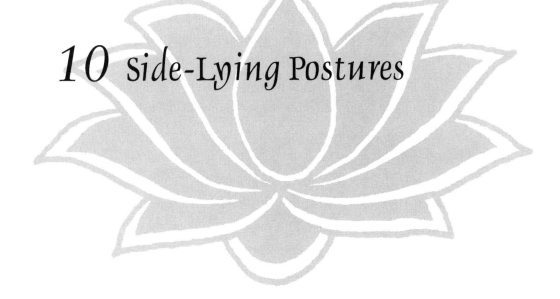

10 Side-Lying Postures

The side position feels wonderful to recipients. This position is especially good for working on people who are pregnant, overweight, or suffer from acute stomachache, as pressure from the abdominal region is released and the body is able to fully relax. It can be an effective compromise for people who are unable to comfortably lie on their backs for prolonged periods of time due to back problems. The side position is also good for reaching the sen lines on the lateral side of the arms, buttocks, and legs. In Thailand side-lying is often used as the principle position for receiving a full-body massage.

The practitioner must pay particular attention to maintaining the recipient's proper alignment when working with the side-lying postures. Proper care should be taken to prop the body so the recipient doesn't slump to one side. Support the receiver's head with a pillow so the cervical spine remains straight. Similarly, a pillow under the bent leg will help keep the lumbar spine straight.

Another key factor to working in the side position is the stability of the practitioner. Each time you apply a side-lying posture reassess the recipient's alignment as well as your own. I have often observed that students may compromise the proper use of stances in the side-lying position because they are focusing on maintaining the stability of the recipient. Do not sacrifice your own stability and sense of center during this section of the massage.

When working with the side-lying postures, perform all of the poses on one side first and then walk to the other side of the recipient to repeat the movements.

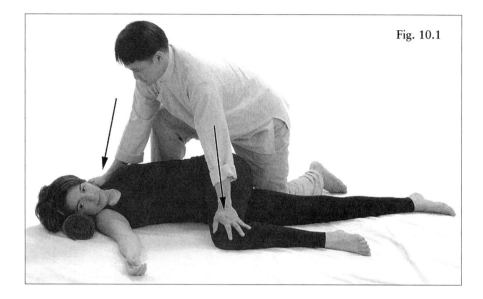

Fig. 10.1

† Dragon Twist

In the Warrior stance, place your right hand on the recipient's left shoulder and your left hand on her left knee.

Gently lean in, gradually applying your body-weight toward the earth, stretching the recipient's knee and shoulder away from one another to give a good spinal twist (**fig. 10.1**).

Benefits: Stretches and lengthens the sympathetic nerve chain; aids digestion and elimination.

Precaution: Do not use jerky movements. Avoid this posture if the recipient has osteoporosis or spinal problems.

Recommended for: Vata, pitta, and kapha

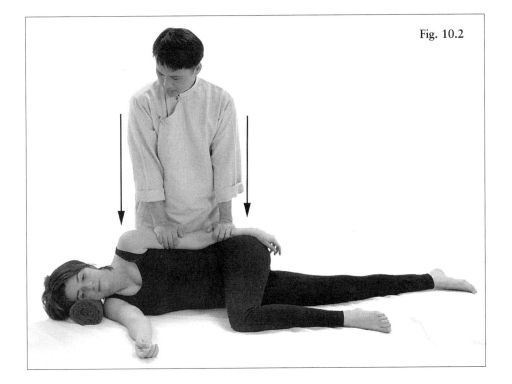

Fig. 10.2

✝ Palming the Arm

Straighten the recipient's left arm and lay it on her side. Move into the Kneeling Diamond stance, with your thighs supporting the recipient's back. Lean in with your bodyweight and palm with both hands on the lateral side of the arm using the forward rocking technique (**fig. 10.2**). Start at the elbow and palm your way toward the wrist and shoulder. With one hand on the wrist and the other on the shoulder, spread the wrist and shoulder away from each other to provide traction to the arm.

Benefits: Compresses the muscles governing the shoulder joint and the extensor muscles governing the wrist, hand, and fingers; relieves tension, especially in the upper arm (this tension is always connected to the back of the shoulder); enhances mobility in the wrist, hand, and fingers.

Common mistake: Not using your thighs to support the recipient's body. Don't be shy about getting close to the recipient's back.

Recommended for: Vata

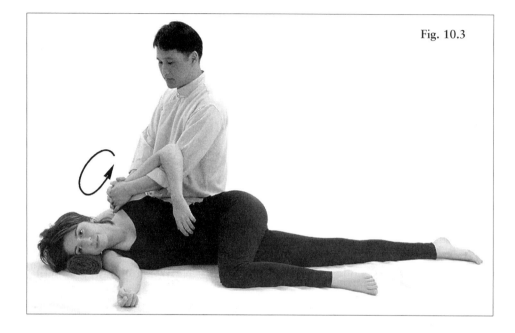

Fig. 10.3

✝ Shoulder Rotation

Sit in the Diamond stance close to the recipient's scapula. Interlace your fingers and wrap them around the recipient's shoulder.

Rotate the shoulder using whirlpool rock (**fig. 10.3**).

Benefits: Relieves tension and increases range of motion in the scapula and shoulder.

Common mistake: The recipient's arm is not relaxed. Don't let the recipient slap herself in the face as her arm is rotating.

Recommended for: Kapha, and for vata if done gently

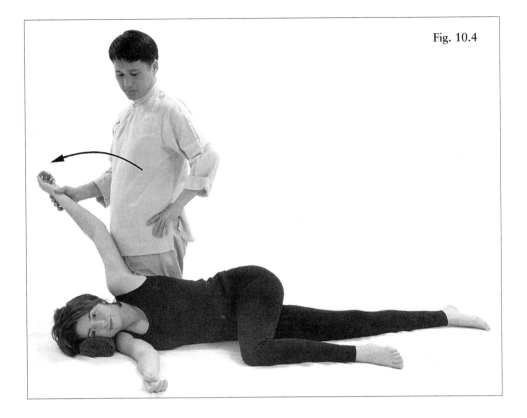

Fig. 10.4

✝ Devil Stretch

Move into the Kneeling Diamond stance with your thighs close to the top of the recipient's scapula. Grasp the recipient's wrist and raise her arm straight up.

Gradually pull the arm across your chest (**fig. 10.4**). The trick is finding the right angle and position to give the recipient's pectoral muscle a good stretch. This is called the Devil Stretch because it is very powerful, so take it easy. Don't overstretch!

Adaptation: For a deeper stretch, lean into the recipient while pulling the arm.

Benefits: Increases range of motion in the scapula and shoulder; stretches the pectoral muscle.

Common mistake: Not finding the right angle to maximize the stretch. It helps to find an angle that provides maximum traction.

Recommended for: Kapha

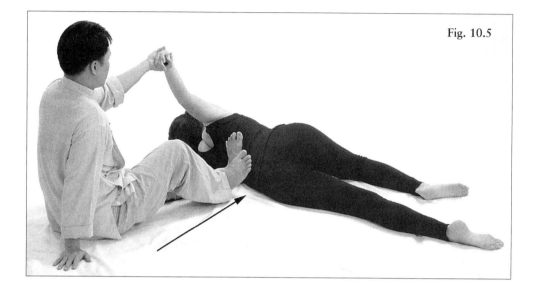

Fig. 10.5

✝ Back Pedal

While maintaining your hold on the recipient's wrist sit down and, with bent legs, place the soles of your feet on the recipient's back. Use your free hand to brace yourself on the mat.

Massage the recipient's back with your feet as if you are pedaling a bicycle, moving from the lower back to the upper back (**fig. 10.5**).

Benefits: Massages the paravertebral muscles; this movement is particularly beneficial for pregnant women.

Precaution: Do not pull the recipient's arm. Be careful not to exert pressure directly on the spine.

Recommended for: Vata and pitta

✝ Standing Side Arc

Grasp the recipient's wrist and ankle and shift from sitting to standing (**fig. 10.6**). Walk backward, giving a gentle stretch to the recipient's thigh (**fig. 10.7**).

When you feel resistance, stop walking and place your foot on the buttock, fixing it in position. Pull the leg by leaning back, providing flexion to the spine and stretching the thigh (**fig. 10.8**). The more beautiful and rounded the body arc is, the more successful the stretch becomes.

Gently release the arm and leg and roll her onto her other side.

Benefits: Stretches the body from hand to foot; particularly beneficial for the stretch to the iliopsoas muscle complex, the deep muscles that connect the spine to the pelvis and thigh; increases flexibility to the midtrunk; tonifies internal organs and assists digestion.

Precaution: Fix your foot firmly on the recipient's buttocks, but do not apply pressure!

Recommended for: Kapha

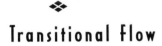

Transitional Flow

Once you have completed the side-lying postures on both sides of the body, place the recipient's arms above her head and then walk toward her feet. In the Archer stance, straighten her bent leg. Hold on to that foot and gently turn the recipient over onto her belly.

This concludes the side-lying postures. We're now ready to move on to the back-position postures.

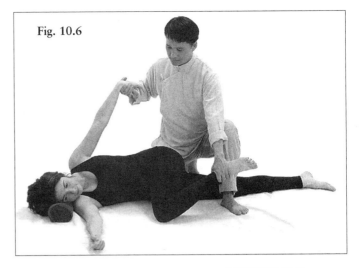

Fig. 10.6

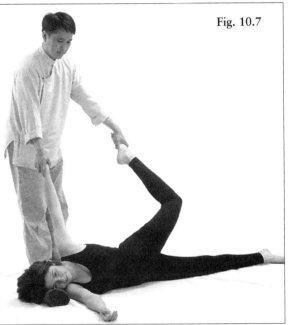

Fig. 10.7

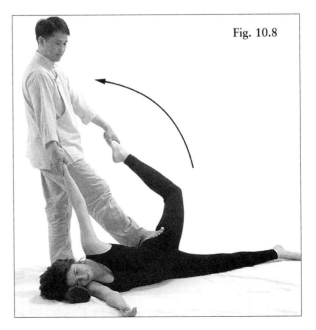

Fig. 10.8

11 Back-Position Postures

Work on the back is in high demand by people in need of a massage. The back is a most pleasurable area on which to receive bodywork, and most massage to this area is highly beneficial for the body. The receiver never seems to have enough of the back massage, so you may want to spend more time on this area. Oftentimes, when I initially come into contact with the recipient's back during a massage, a sigh of relief escapes that seems to say, "Finally, someone is helping me release this tension!"

In this chapter you will be introduced to various palming and thumbing variations to stimulate the flow of energy along the sen lines of the back. Use the induced breathing technique of falling into the recipient on the exhalation; this promotes deep breathing and the intake of re-energizing prana.

At this point in the Thai Yoga Massage session many recipients will be deeply relaxed; some may even be close to falling asleep. You might want to have towels or small pillows available to tuck under the recipient's ankles, upper chest, and lower abdomen, all for the purpose of relaxing the lower back. Placing a pillow under the recipient's forehead will keep the nose from being pushed into the floor. If the recipient's head is turned to one side, ask her to periodically move her head to the other side to avoid stiffness in the neck.

With the exception of the Sanuk and Locust poses, all the back-position postures are performed bilaterally.

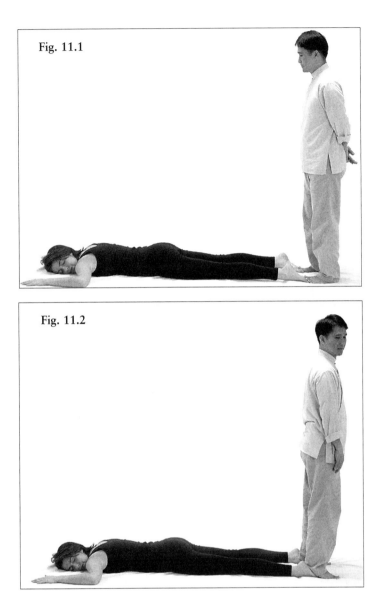

Fig. 11.1

Fig. 11.2

Sole Walk

Adjust the recipient's feet so the toes are pointing inward toward each other. Slowly walk on the feet, moving from the small toe up to the instep and back down to the toes (**fig. 11.1 and 11.2**).

Adaptation: If you have trouble balancing, try walking on one foot at a time. With practice this movement will become easy.

Benefits: Compresses the intrinsic muscles of the foot; flexes the Achilles tendon; provides a reflexology massage to the feet, relieving tension and stiffness and stimulating organs and body systems.

Precaution: Avoid walking on the ball of the foot. Be careful not to crush the toes. If the recipient's foot should cramp, have her rotate the foot until it is at ease and then proceed with the massage.

Recommended for: Vata, pitta, and kapha

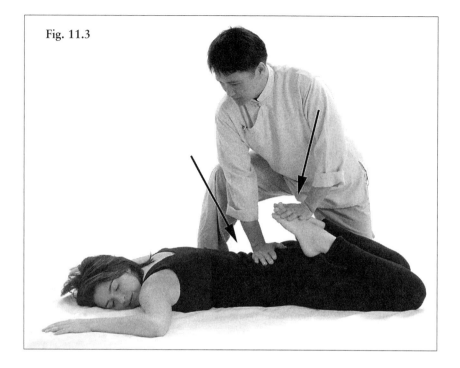

Fig. 11.3

Thunderbolt

Move into the Warrior stance and position your-self on the side of the recipient. Hold the dorsal side of the feet with your left hand and bring the legs toward the buttocks.

When the knees reach 90 degrees, place your right hand on the recipient's lower back, just above the sacrum. Press gradually but firmly downward toward the mat and slightly feet-ward. Bend the recipient's legs the rest of the way toward the buttocks, pressing the feet down toward the mat and slightly head-ward (**fig. 11.3**). Use your bodyweight to apply appropri-ate pressure.

Adaptation: If your hands are small or the recip-ient's feet are big, place one foot on top of the other for easier control.

Benefits: Provides lumbar-sacral extension; relieves lower back tension and constipation; tonifies the kidneys; stretches the quadriceps and iliopsoas muscles.

Common mistake: The hand does not fix the sacrum firmly enough, causing pinching in the lower back. Be sure to use your bodyweight to maintain a firm hold on the sacrum.

Precaution: Proceed gently if the recipient has spinal or lower back problems.

Recommended for: Vata

Sanuk

This excellent position for working on the buttocks must be the ultimate favorite of traditional Thai masseurs. It is a bit tricky to perfect the transition, so practice, practice, practice. (In Thailand you often find not-so-serious practitioners doing the Sanuk while smoking, drinking whiskey, and gossiping with fellow masseurs. This is the kind of contradiction that one may encounter while traveling to Thailand to practice Thai Yoga Massage, so it is important to study at the right source. For more information on massage schools in Thailand see the resources on page 142.)

Scoop the recipient's left knee with your left hand, bending the leg to 90 degrees and coming into the Archer stance near her knees (**fig. 11.4**). Place your free hand beside her right hip for stability. In one fluid motion, lift the leg and glide your right thigh underneath (**fig. 11.5**). Be careful not to jam your knee into the recipient's groin as you glide into position.

Sit down in a comfortable position with the recipient's leg resting across your thighs. Forward rock and roll with the forearm on the back, buttocks, and legs (**fig. 11.6**). Use your elbows for deep stimulation to the buttocks. Gently slide your leg out from underneath the recipient's leg and place her leg on the mat. Proceed to the Locust pose, or repeat the Sanuk pose on the other side.

Benefits: Forearm roll on the gluteus maximus and gluteus medius eases sciatic pain; relieves tension around sciatic muscles; relieves tired legs and tension in the buttocks.

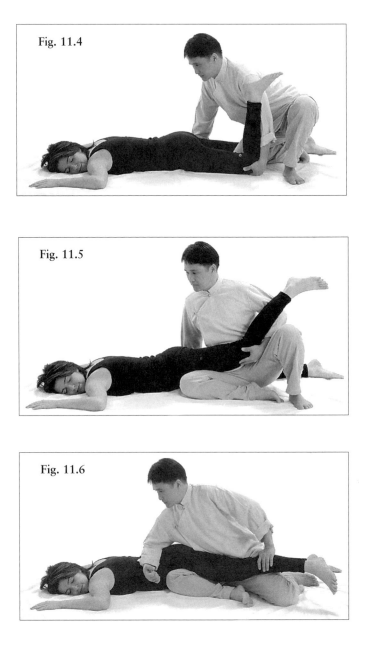

Fig. 11.4

Fig. 11.5

Fig. 11.6

Common mistake: The practitioner does not slide in close enough to the recipient's hip.

Recommended for: Vata and pitta

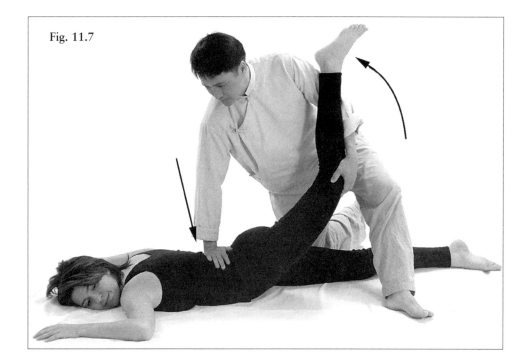

Fig. 11.7

† Locust

This pose is best suited to people who are flexible. You want to avoid this posture if the recipient has lower back problems.

In the Warrior stance raise the recipient's left leg, holding it at the knee with your left hand. Fix your free hand on the recipient's lower back, just above the sacrum. Apply gentle pressure toward the floor.

Using your bodyweight, lean your torso toward the recipient's upper back (**fig. 11.7**). The recipient will receive a deep stretch along the front of the thigh and into the hip joint.

Gently lower the leg. Repeat the Sanuk and Locust poses on the other side.

Benefits: Stretches the quadriceps and iliopsoas muscles and the abdomen; helps prevent hernia; strengthens the abdominal muscles and massages the internal organs.

Common mistake: Practitioner does not use his leg to support the hand that is holding the recipient's knee. This is an important safeguard in the event that the practitioner's hand slips.

Recommended for: Kapha, and for vata if done gently

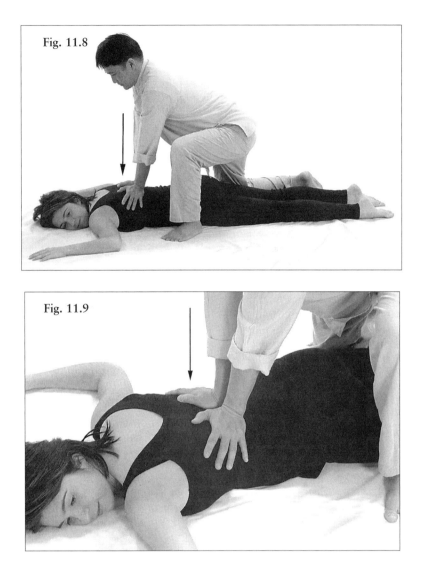

Fig. 11.8

Fig. 11.9

Palming Sen on the Back

Straddle the recipient in the Warrior stance. With arms and back straight, palm up and down the back on either side of the spine (**fig. 11.8**).

Use your bodyweight to fall into the recipient (**fig. 11.9**). Synchronize your breath as you forward rock, and encourage the dance of Thai Yoga Massage to emerge.

Ask the recipient to move her head from side to side every few minutes to prevent stiffness in the neck. In total, the palming should take about five to ten minutes for the basic massage and ten to twenty minutes for the extended massage.

Benefits: Works on the paravertebral muscles and autonomic nervous system; relieves back stress and muscle spasms; stimulates the internal organs; aligns the spine.

Precaution: Be careful not to put pressure directly on the spine. With pregnant women, work the sen in a side-lying or a sitting position.

Recommended for: Vata, pitta, and kapha

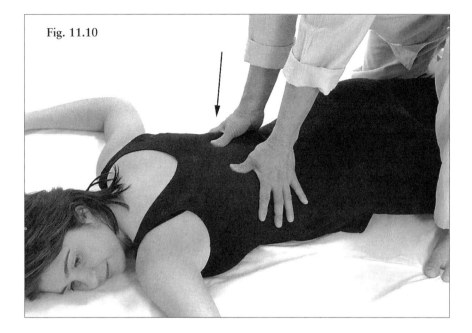

Fig. 11.10

Thumbing Sen on Back

Still in the Warrior stance, thumb up and down the back on either side of the spine (**fig. 11.10**). Make sure your arms and back are straight. Use your bodyweight to fall in to the recipient's body.

Synchronize your breath as you forward rock, allowing the thumbing to become a dance.

As with palming on the back, do not put pressure directly on the spine. Ask the recipient to move her head from side to side every five minutes to prevent a stiff neck from developing.

Benefits: Works on the paravertebral muscles and autonomic nervous system; relieves back stress and muscle spasms; stimulates the internal organs; aligns the spine.

Precaution: With pregnant women, work the sen in a side-lying or a sitting position.

Recommended for: Vata, pitta, and kapha

✝ Palming and Thumbing Variations

Here are a few other possibilities for ways to massage your recipient in palming and thumbing.

Twisting Palm

In the Warrior stance, cup the spine with one hand placed over the other. Rock in with your bodyweight and twist the palm on the muscles (**fig. 11.11**). The direction of the twist is inward toward the spine; however, be careful not to put pressure directly on the spine.

Circulating Palm

In the Warrior stance, move your palm in a circular motion up and down the muscles beside the spine (**fig. 11.12**).

Double Palm Pressure

In the Kneeling Diamond stance, place the heels of your hands on the ridge of the spinal muscles. With arms and back straight, fall in with your bodyweight and palm up and down the back (**fig. 11.13**).

This is one of the more powerful palming techniques.

Double Thumb Pressure

In the Kneeling Diamond stance, place thumb on top of thumb on the recipient's spinal muscles. With arms and back straight, fall in with your bodyweight to tonify the sen lines on the back (**fig. 11.14**).

This is a powerful thumbing technique.

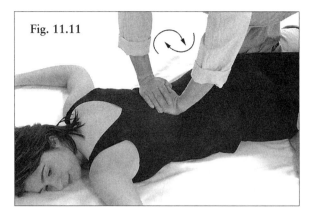

Fig. 11.11

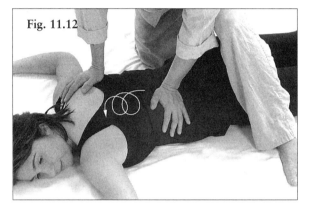

Fig. 11.12

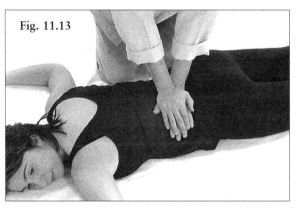

Fig. 11.13

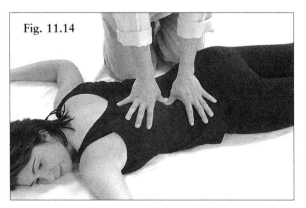

Fig. 11.14

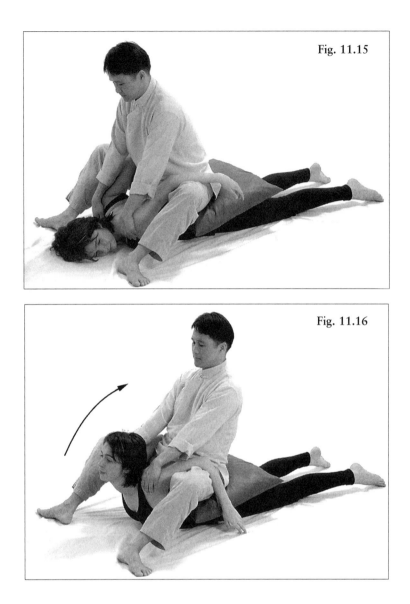

Fig. 11.15

Fig. 11.16

Pillow Cobra

From palming and thumbing along the back, place a pillow on the recipient's lower back. Gently sit on the recipient's sacrum with your feet flat on the floor. Place the recipient's arms across your thighs, with her hands hanging to the side. Grasp the recipient's shoulders from above (**fig. 11.15**).

Using directed breathing, ask the recipient to inhale deeply, then exhale. On the exhale, lean back, using your bodyweight to lift the recipient into a backbend (**fig. 11.16**).

Release by gently returning the recipient's chest to the mat. Ask that she turn her head to the side as she comes back down to the mat.

Benefits: Flexes the spine; opens the chest; relieves lower back ache and spinal stiffness.

Common mistake: Practitioner's feet are too close together, causing instability in the posture.

Precaution: Avoid jerky movements.

Recommended for: Vata and pitta

† Classic Cobra

From the Pillow Cobra, move back into the Kneeling Diamond stance with your knees fixed on the recipient's buttocks. Ask the recipient to hold on to your wrists or forearms (**fig. 11.17**).

Using directed breathing, ask the recipient to inhale deeply, then exhale. On the exhale lean backward, using the leverage of the movement to gently pull the recipient into a backbend (**fig. 11.18**).

Release by returning to an upright kneeling position, gently returning the recipient to the mat.

Benefits: Flexes the spine; provides traction through the shoulder girdle, stretching the deltoid muscles; opens the chest; stimulates the internal organs; aids digestion; promotes flexibility of spine; relieves lower back ache and spinal stiffness; relieves nasal congestion.

Common mistake: Practitioner's grip of the wrist or forearm is not secure. Knees are not firmly on the buttocks. Be sure to position yourself strongly and securely before performing this posture.

Precaution: Avoid performing this posture with recipients who have dislocated a shoulder.

Recommended for: Kapha

❖

Transitional Flow

Place the recipient's arms above her head, palms facing down. In the Kneeling Diamond stance, hold on to one foot and pull her leg toward you, maintaining traction. Gradually turn the recipient's foot, gently rotating her torso to bring her into the supine position.

This is the end of the back-position postures. We're now ready to move on to the double-leg postures.

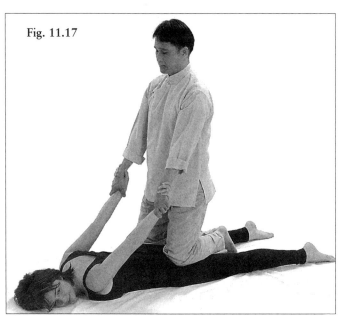

Fig. 11.17

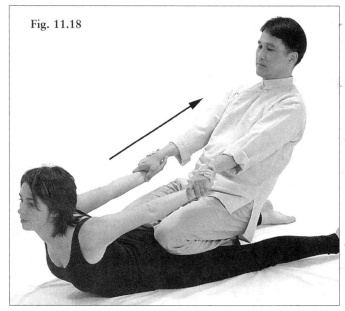

Fig. 11.18

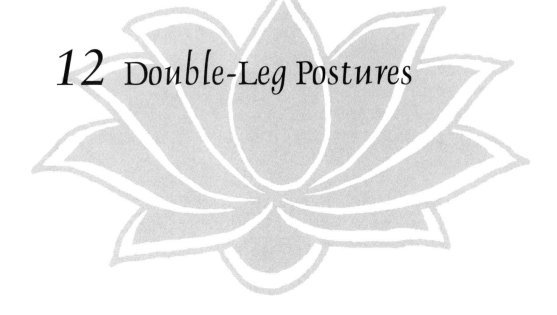

12 Double-Leg Postures

Since two legs are heavier to lift than one, the first thing we should address when preparing to lift both legs is how to use the body sensibly. When shifting between sitting and standing positions it is advisable that the practitioner moves deliberately, paying attention to proper body mechanics so that you do not harm your lower back. For example, when you come to standing first shift your body into the Diamond stance, then move into the Warrior stance, and from there come up to stand in the Tai Chi stance.

Another important tenet of good body mechanics in Thai Yoga Massage is to never bend from the hip to lift a recipient's leg or arm. Use your stances to progressively move into a standing position, and lift the legs by using proper body mechanics. After one hundred Thai Yoga Massage sessions your back will be most grateful.

After performing each double-leg posture, walk away from the recipient while holding under her heels to straighten her legs. Once you feel traction through the legs, gently shake out the legs and rock them from side to side. This helps release any residual tension (and it also feels great). Listen for "oohs" and "ahhs." Upon completion of the double-leg sequence, squat or come down to the ground through Warrior stance and place the recipient's legs back on the mat.

All of the double-leg postures are performed bilaterally. Since many of these postures involve placing the recipient in inversions, they should be performed with a clear understanding of contraindications (see chapter 4).

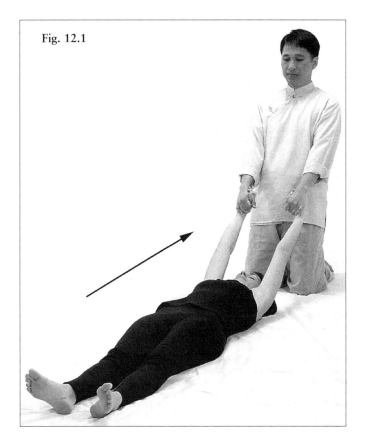

Fig. 12.1

The Long Stretch

Bring the recipient's arms above her head. Grasp her wrists and come into the Kneeling Diamond stance (**fig. 12.1**). Lean back, giving the recipient a long stretch through the arms, torso, hip joints, and legs.

Benefits: Provides traction to the shoulder girdle, stretching the biceps, triceps, and scapulae; increases shoulder mobility; relieves arm and shoulder tension.

Precaution: In cases of previous shoulder dislocation, take care with the amount of traction you provide as there is a danger of a relapse. Be similarly careful with frozen or stiff shoulders.

Recommended for: Pitta

Half-Plough

Move to the recipient's feet and come into the Diamond stance. Hold under the recipient's heels (**fig. 12.2**).

In one fluid motion, move into the Warrior stance while pushing the recipient's legs up toward the ceiling (**fig. 12.3**). The palms of your hands are on the recipient's heels. Keep your arms and back straight.

Keeping your palms on the recipient's heels, stand up into the Tai Chi stance. Rock the recipient's legs forward three times (**fig. 12.4**). To release, slowly walk backward while holding the recipient's feet. Gently shake out the legs and rock them from side to side.

Move on to the Yoke posture for an extended Thai Yoga Massage session. The Yoke is particularly good for recipients who have a stiff back and are generally less flexible. For a basic session, move on to the Butterfly posture.

Benefits: Rolls and massages the paravertebral muscles; tones the thyroid gland; extends the nuchal ligament at the back of the neck; reduces stress on the spinal column, lower back, and back of the neck; benefits internal organs; assists in regulating low blood pressure.

Precaution: Never perform a full Plough pose. Avoid this posture in the event of heart disease or high blood pressure, and during pregnancy or menstruation.

Recommended for: Kapha

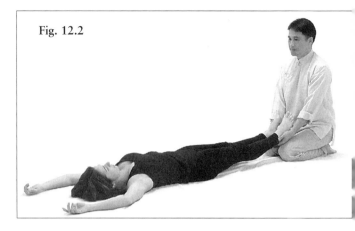

Fig. 12.2

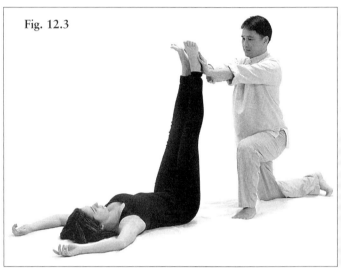

Fig. 12.3

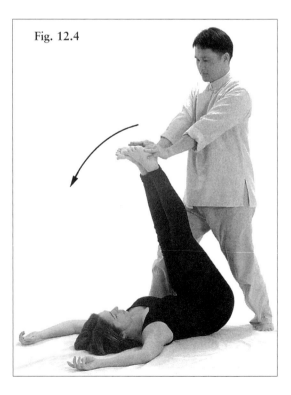

Fig. 12.4

✝ The Yoke

In a Tai Chi stance, bend the recipient's left leg (**fig. 12.5**). Place the left ankle above the right knee. Place the recipient's right leg on your left shoulder (**fig. 12.6**).

Grasp the recipient's bent left ankle. With your free hand, rock forward and palm the hamstrings of the bent left leg (**fig. 12.7**). Direct your palming pressure toward the center of the body.

To release, slowly separate the recipient's legs and walk backward while holding the feet. Gently shake out the legs and rock them from side to side. Repeat the posture on the opposite side.

Adaptation: If you are very tall in relation to the recipient, come down into the Warrior stance after adjusting the legs.

Benefits: Compresses the hamstrings; flexes the hip joints; stimulates the kidneys and intestines; stretches the lower back; helps to relieve constipation.

Precaution: Avoid this posture in case of heart problems or hernia, and during pregnancy.

Recommended for: Vata and pitta

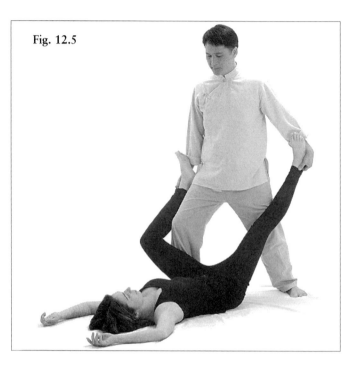

Fig. 12.5

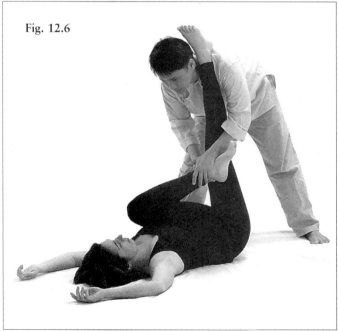

Fig. 12.6

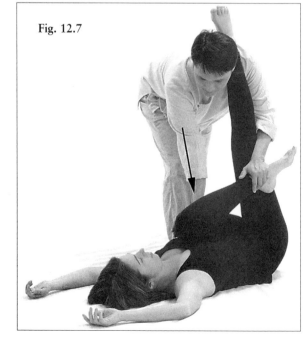

Fig. 12.7

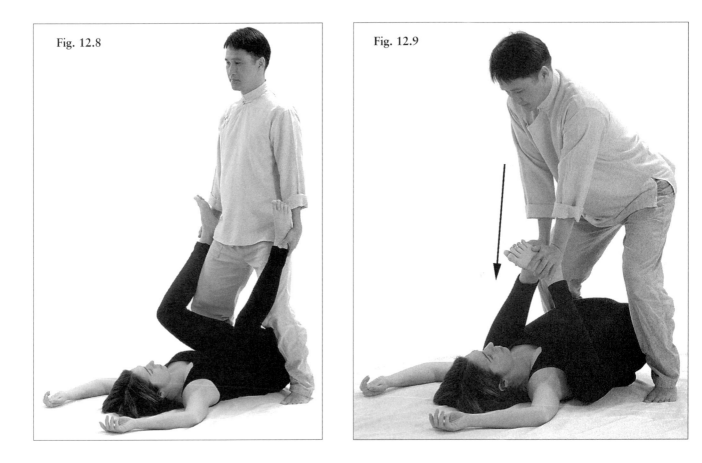

Fig. 12.8

Fig. 12.9

Butterfly

Bend the recipient's legs with the knees hip-distance apart (**fig. 12.8**). Place the soles of the feet together and allow the knees to spread out wide.

Push the feet downward toward the recipient's nose (**fig. 12.9**). Steadily press your body-weight toward the floor through the recipient's feet and legs; be sure not to bounce. To release, walk back while holding the feet. Gently shake out the legs and rock them from side to side.

Benefits: Stretches the adductor, gluteus maximus, and hamstring muscles; opens the hip joints; strengthens the ability to sit, squat, and do floor activities without discomfort; stimulates the internal organs and benefits digestion.

Precaution: Avoid this posture in the event of untreated high blood pressure or heart disease, and during pregnancy.

Recommended for: Pitta and kapha

✝ AG Pose (Anti-Gravitational Spinal Relaxation Pose)

Bend the recipient's legs, knees together. Place the recipient's insteps on your knees. Keep your knees together and your feet spread shoulder-width apart. Reach around and interlace your fingers just above the recipient's knees (**fig. 12.10**). Hold tight!

Pull the recipient's legs firmly toward your body (**fig. 12.11**). With a confident lift and squat, bring the recipient up into the AG pose (**fig. 12.12**).

To release, roll up and return the recipient to the original position. Slowly walk back while holding the feet. Gently shake out the legs and rock them from side to side.

Adaptation: If you have sharp, pointy kneecaps, use a folded towel between your knees and the recipient's insteps. For a more secure grip, use a scarf or a yoga strap.

Benefits: This inversion exercise relaxes the lower back, increases space between the vertebrae, and provides traction to the spine; this is one of the most surprising and well-loved poses.

Common mistake: The practitioner does not stand with his knees together, and/or stands too far away from the recipient to do the posture effectively. It is easier to execute this pose when you are closer to the recipient, but it's a fine balance. Don't be intimidated by this posture; it's easier than it looks. Just keep your knees together, gauge your distance from the recipient, remember to breathe, and—whatever you do—don't let go!

Precaution: Do not lift the recipient's neck off the mat. To be safe, advise the recipient to tuck her chin to her chest when releasing the pose.

Recommended for: Pitta and kapha

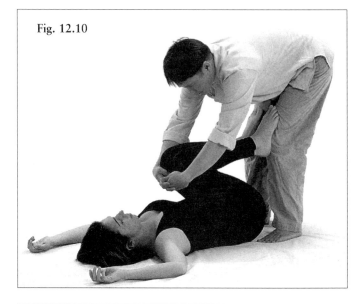
Fig. 12.10

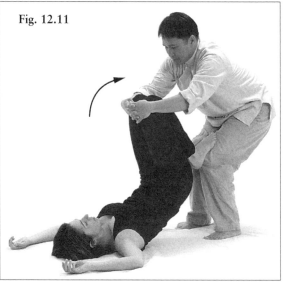
Fig. 12.11

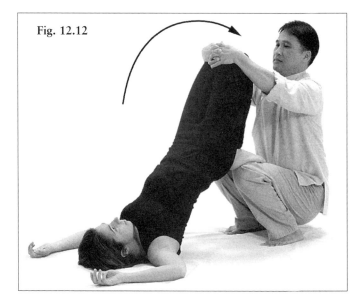
Fig. 12.12

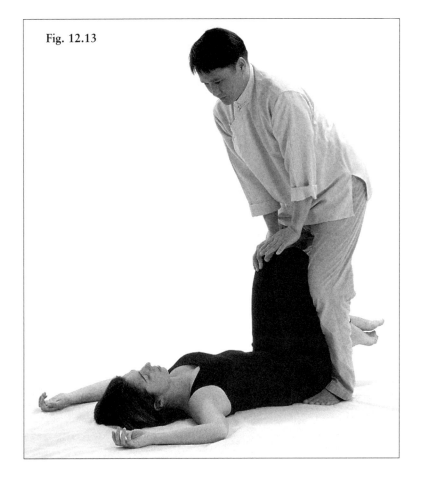

Fig. 12.13

Hip-Hop

Bend the recipient's legs, bringing the knees together and sandwiching them between your legs. Tuck your feet underneath the recipient's buttocks. Keeping your back and arms straight, alternately palm the recipient's knees using the bamboo rock, pressing the lower back and sacrum toward the mat (**fig. 12.13**).

Release the posture by pushing the knees toward the recipient's chest. Rest the recipient's insteps on your knees and then walk back while holding the feet. Gently shake out the legs and rock them from side to side.

Benefits: Compresses the sacrum and hip joints; relieves lower back stress; tones the kidneys. This pose is another all-time favorite.

Recommended for: Vata

Yoga Mudra

Bend the recipient's legs, crossing them at the ankles and placing them below your knees (**fig. 12.14**). Direct the feet toward the floor and align your shin bones with the recipient's thighs. Ask the recipient to hold on to your wrists or forearms (**fig. 12.15**).

Pull the recipient away from the ground by straightening your legs. Using your bodyweight, push inward toward the recipient's body with your knees (**fig. 12.16**). This will bring the recipient's legs close to her torso. Make sure to use your bodyweight, not your arm strength, to execute this posture.

To release, allow the recipient to gently fall back to the mat. Uncross her legs and walk back holding the feet. Gently shake out the legs and rock them from side to side.

Adaptation: If necessary, place a cushion between your shin bones and the recipient to avoid bone-on-bone contact, which can be painful.

Benefits: Provides traction to the shoulder girdle; flexes the hip adductors. This exercise is a good complement to any backbend.

Precaution: Proceed with caution if the recipient's knees are sore or recently injured.

Recommended for: Pitta

❖

Transitional Flow

Lower the recipient onto her back and let her hands fall to her sides. Hold on to her heels and straighten her legs while walking back. Gently lower her legs.

As a possible modification, bring the legs together and support the heels with one hand while moving into the Warrior stance. With your free hand, place a pillow under the recipient's knees and gently lower her legs. This will lift the recipient's knees, relaxing her spine; for female recipients, it also reduces pressure on the ovaries.

This is the end of the double-leg postures. We're now ready to move on to the abdomen, chest, arm, and hand postures.

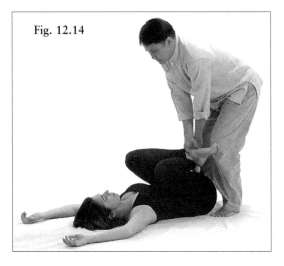

Fig. 12.14

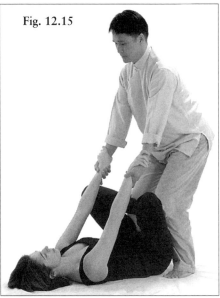

Fig. 12.15

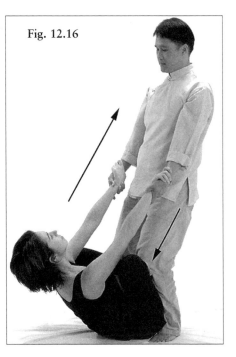

Fig. 12.16

13 Abdomen, Chest, Arm, and Hand Postures

The abdomen contains our organs of digestion and elimination and, for that reason, can be a very sensitive part of the body. Some people can be shy about being touched in this area, so first ask your recipient if she would like to be massaged here.

Begin by gently rubbing and soothing the abdomen. Follow the breath of the recipient and calmly synchronize your movement to this flow. When you feel the recipient is relaxed, lightly apply pressure on the five organ-reflex points (**Fig. 13.1**). Do not massage or touch the breasts. If the recipient has eaten immediately prior to your session, place the abdominal work at the end of the session, just before the facial massage. Be sure to avoid massaging the abdomen if the recipient is pregnant or has an intense stomachache. Instead, a longer massage on the back, on the side, or in the sitting position is recommended.

For the basic Thai Yoga Massage follow the techniques outlined below for Abdominal Massage 1; for the extended version proceed with Abdominal Massage 2. You can sit on either side of recipient for the abdominal massage.

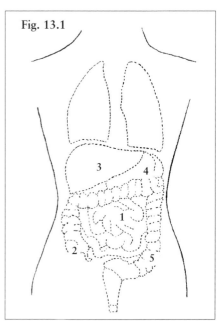

Fig. 13.1

Organ reflex points for Abdominal Massage 1

1 = Small intestine   4 = Spleen and stomach
2 = Ascending colon   5 = Descending colon
3 = Liver

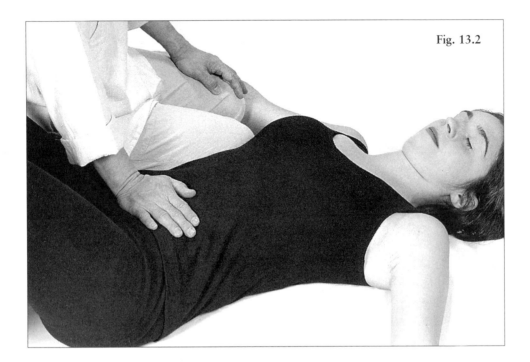

Fig. 13.2

Abdominal Massage 1

Lay a Brick

When I was a little boy my mother would place a brick on my abdomen to calm my hyperactive disposition. Putting pressure on the abdominal area encourages deep breathing and has a very calming effect.

Sit in the Diamond stance alongside the recip-ient. Place your hand over the area just below the recipient's belly button and synchronize your breath with hers (**fig. 13.2**).

With a straight arm, rock in gently with your bodyweight on an exhalation and ease off on the inhalation.

Sun-Moon Stroke

Sit in the Diamond stance alongside the recipient. Following the direction of the large intestine, circle one hand in a clockwise manner around the perimeter of the abdomen. This represents the sun.

The other hand follows in the same direction at the same pace, but lifts off the abdomen as the sun stroke continues circulating (**fig. 13.3**). This half-circle stroke represents the moon.

This stroke has a very soothing effect in preparation for palming.

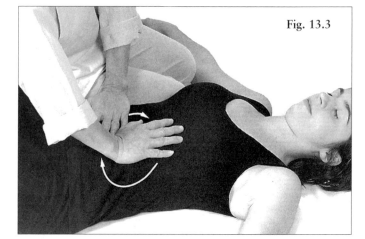

Fig. 13.3

Palming

From the Diamond stance, place your palm on organ-reflex point 1 (**fig. 13.4**). Wait for an exhalation and rock in gently with your bodyweight. Hold for one full inhale and exhale, and ease off with the next inhalation.

Repeat on points 2 through 5.

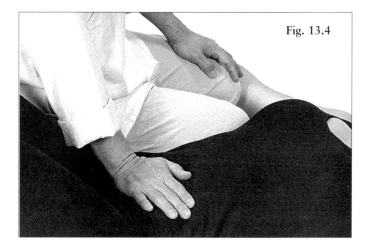

Fig. 13.4

Finger Pressing

From the Diamond stance, place the fingers of both hands on organ-reflex point 1 (**fig. 13.5**).

Wait for an exhalation and rock in gently with your bodyweight. Don't push in sharply with your fingertips; simply ease in with your fingers and ease off with the inhalation. Repeat on points 2 through 5.

Repeat the Sun-Moon stroke to end this part of the session.

Benefits of Abdominal Massage 1: Releases tension in the belly; helps to relieve constipation, as working in the clockwise direction assists with elimination.

Precaution: Do not press strongly on recipients with heart disease.

Recommended for: Vata, pitta, and kapha

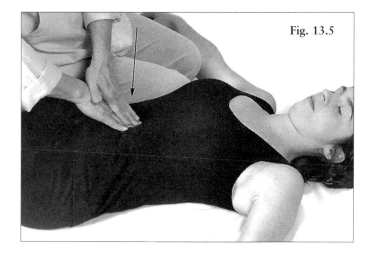

Fig. 13.5

✝ Abdominal Massage 2

For a deeper experience, continue the abdominal massage with the following strokes. Avoid these strokes during pregnancy or acute stomachache.

Circular Pressure on Organ Reflex Points

Sit in the Diamond stance alongside the recipient with your fingers on organ-reflex point 1. As the recipient exhales, fall in with your bodyweight and circulate clockwise (**fig. 13.6**). Don't push in sharply with your fingertips; just ease in with the full length of your fingers. Ease off with the recipient's inhalation.

Repeat on all eleven organ-reflex points (**fig. 13.7**).

Energy Ball

From the Diamond stance alongside the recipient, tuck one hand under the back, palm up. Place the second hand on top of the abdomen.

Imagine cupping a ball of energy between both hands. Massage by pushing, pulling, rotating, and playing with the energy ball (**fig. 13.8**).

Benefits of Abdominal Massage 2: Releases tension in the belly; stimulates the bowels. If the recipient is constipated work longer on the recipient's left side, around the area of the descending colon.

Precaution: Do not press strongly on recipients with heart disease.

Recommended for: Vata, pitta, and kapha

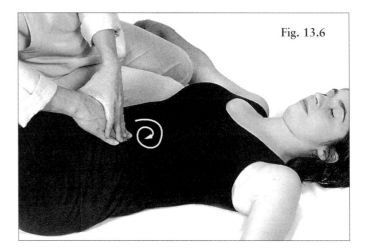

Fig. 13.6

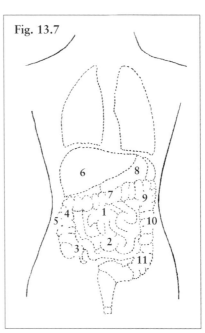

Fig. 13.7

Organ reflex points for Abdominal Massage 2

1, 2 = Navel and small intestine
3, 4 = Ascending colon
5 = Kidneys
6 = Liver
7 = Transverse colon
8 = Spleen and stomach
9 = Descending colon
10 = Kidneys
11 = Descending colon

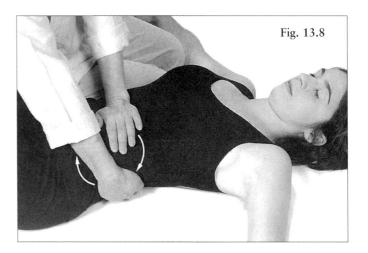

Fig. 13.8

Abdominal Massage (Alternative Posture)

As an alternative to the Diamond stance I recommend the following posture. It is very effective for giving an abdominal massage, but it is also very intimate. Therefore, I advise that you only do it with recipients you know well.

Sit in the Diamond stance at the feet of the recipient and place your hands under the feet. In one fluid motion, move into the Kneeling Diamond stance while pushing the recipient's legs upward (**fig. 13.9**). Keep your arms and back straight. The palms of your hands should be on the recipient's heels.

Continue pushing the legs up as you walk in with your knees. Move in close, your knees against the recipient's lower back (**fig. 13.10**).

Allow the legs to fall on either side of your hips while your thighs support the recipient's lower back. The abdomen is now close to yours and very accessible to your hands (**fig. 13.11**).

Forearm rolling and two palming variations are particularly effective from this posture.

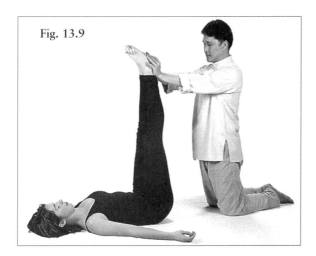

Fig. 13.9

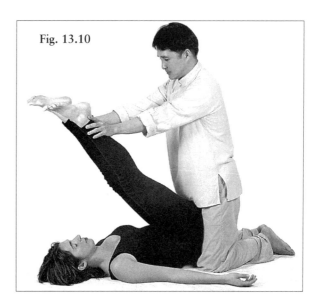

Fig. 13.10

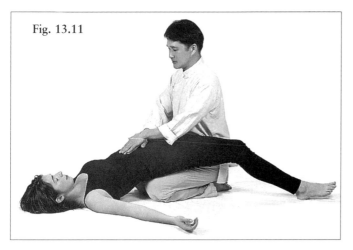

Fig. 13.11

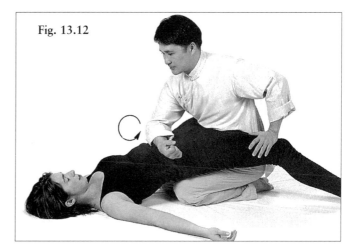

Fig. 13.12

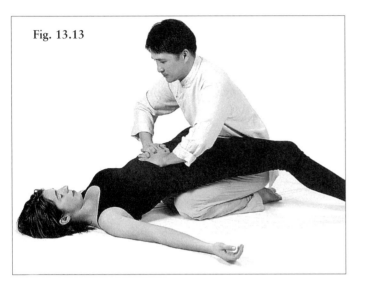

Fig. 13.13

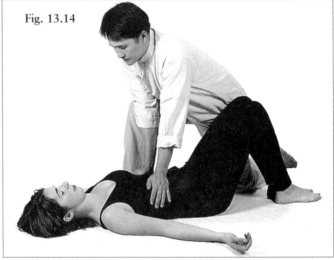

Fig. 13.14

Forearm Rolling

Place your forearm on the recipient's belly. Forward rock as you roll your forearm up and down the abdomen (**fig. 13.12**).

Hand Waves

Interlace your fingers and place both hands on the recipient's abdomen, palms down. Move your hands in a side-to-side motion, like waves on the ocean (**fig. 13.13**).

Opening the Chest

Position yourself in the Warrior stance beside the recipient. Place your hands on the ribs, with the heels of the hands facing the middle of the chest. The fingers follow the ribs along the side of rib cage (**fig. 13.14**).

Beginning just above the floating ribs, fall in with your bodyweight on an exhalation, spreading the chest. Ease off on the next inhalation. Move slightly upward on the rib cage and repeat.

Move to the upper chest and apply a third time just below the shoulders.

Benefits: Expansion of the chest and compression of the costal cartilage maintains flexibility through the rib cage; relieves chest tension.

Precaution: Spread your weight out evenly between your palms. Avoid pressing on the breasts. Do not perform this posture on recipients with osteoporosis.

Recommended for: Kapha

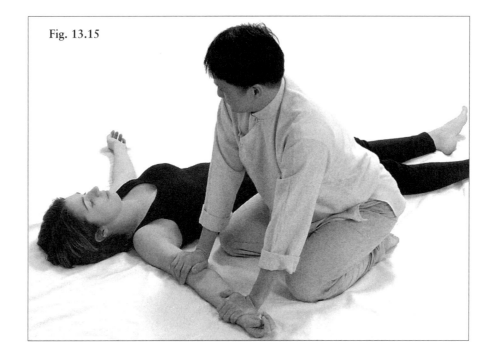

Fig. 13.15

Palming Sen on Arms

Sit alongside the recipient in the Open Diamond stance. Raise the recipient's arm to a 90-degree angle from the body. Place one hand on the recipient's wrist and the other hand above the crook of the elbow (**fig. 13.15**).

Palm up and down the recipient's arm using bamboo rocking, one hand moving from the wrist to the elbow and the other from the elbow to just below the underarm. Move on to Thumbing Sen on the same arm.

Benefits: Tones the brachial, ulnar, and radial arteries; compresses along the intraosseous sheath in the forearm; clears lactic acid and relieves fatigue and numbness in the arms.

Precaution: Avoid pressing on bones and the underarm.

Recommended for: Vata, pitta, and kapha

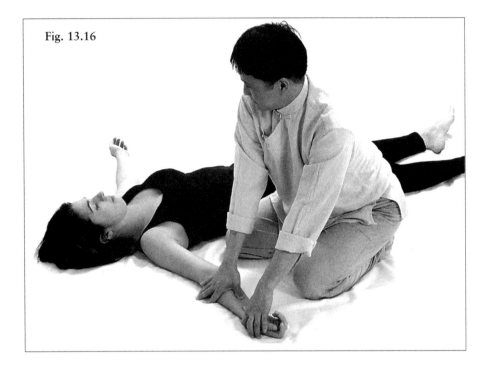

Fig. 13.16

Thumbing Sen on Arms

Continuing to sit alongside the recipient in the Open Diamond stance, use the thumb-chasing-thumb method to palpate the sen from the wrist to the elbow and back to the wrist (**fig. 13.16**). Then palpate from the elbow to just below the underarm and return. This movement is best executed by bamboo rocking.

If you are performing a basic Thai Yoga Massage session, repeat Palming Sen on this arm, move on to Hand Massage, and then move to the other side of the recipient's body and repeat the arm-massage sequence, beginning with Palming Sen. If you're performing an extended session, repeat Palming Sen on this arm, move on to Blood Stop and Hand Massage, and then perform the entire sequence on the other side.

Benefits: Stimulates the sen lines; relieves tightness and numbness in the arms and hands.

Precaution: Avoid pressing on the bones and the underarm.

Recommended for: Vata, pitta, and kapha

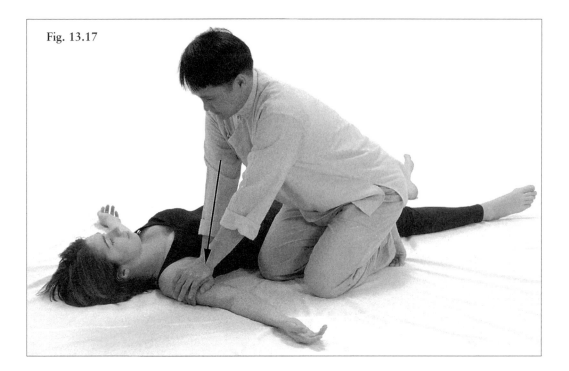

Fig. 13.17

✝ Blood Stop on Arms

Move in to the Cat 3 stance. Place your hands on the biceps close to the armpit and apply direct pressure (**fig. 13.17**). This will compress the brachial artery and restrict blood flow into the arm.

Hold the pressure for 25 seconds and release. The receiver should feel a tingling sensation rushing through her arm to the fingers.

Benefits: Compresses the brachial arteries, the main supplier of blood to the hands. This sudden flow of blood cleans the blood vessels of dead cells and improves circulation.

Precaution: Avoid doing this movement with people who have hypertension or heart problems, and on people who are overweight.

Recommended for: Kapha

Hand Massage

Another all-time favorite Thai massage move is the hand massage. A lot of people work with their hands—at the computer, doing carpentry, cooking, writing, massaging, and so on.

For a wonderful hand massage, begin at the wrist. Let the recipient's hand rest in your palms and massage the wrist with your thumbs (**fig. 13.18**). Then interlace your ring and index fingers with the recipient's fingers, spreading and stretching the recipient's palm (**fig. 13.19**). Use your thumbs to massage the palm.

Next, gently squeeze and pull the fingers one by one (**fig. 13.20**). Then squeeze around the entire hand (**fig. 13.21**).

To finish, gently stroke the hand and lay it down softly (**fig. 13.22**).

Benefits: Relieves tension and arthritis in the

hand; increases mobility of the hand; stimulates the numerous acupressure points on the hand.

Recommended for: Vata, pitta, and kapha

❖

Transitional Flow

Sit comfortably in a cross-legged position a few inches behind the recipient's head in preparation for the face massage. We're now ready to move on to the session's close.

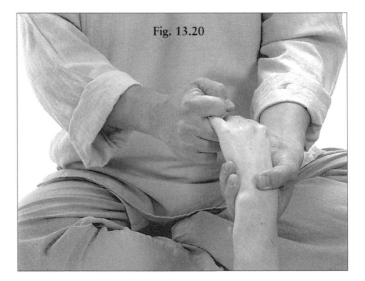

Fig. 13.20

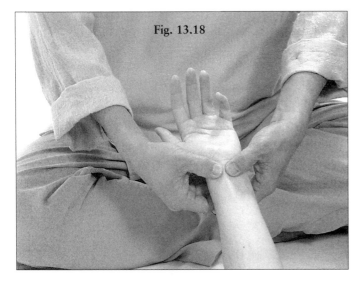

Fig. 13.18

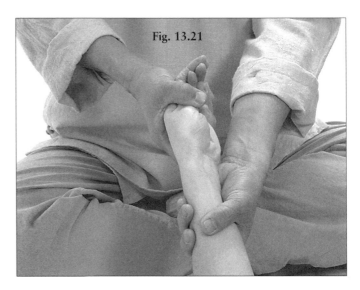

Fig. 13.21

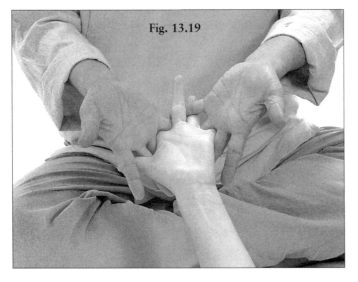

Fig. 13.19

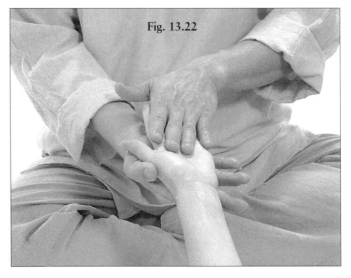

Fig. 13.22

14 Session Closure

Once you arrive at the session closure you have danced your way through a beautiful massage. However, the best is yet to come: the face massage. Whatever mistakes you may have made during a session, you will be forgiven by providing the recipient with a good face massage.

The facial techniques of a traditional Thai massage are chopping, squeezing, pinching, and slapping; however, ending a session this way shocks the body and mind of most Western recipients. This is not a very relaxed way to end a massage. The Lotus Palm approach to Thai Yoga Massage provides an alternative to the abrupt method offered in Thailand. We finish with a gentle rubbing and stroking of the facial muscles. Keeping with the tradition of working the acupressure points, we still include light circulation of pressure points with the fingers. Following the face massage, finish as you began: with a moment of silence in Namaskar.

When beginning the massage, move in slowly and gently with your hands so as not to startle the recipient. At the end, remove your hands slowly and gently.

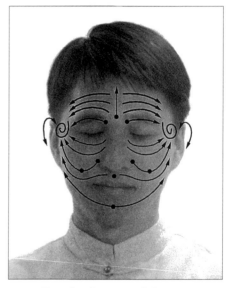

Follow the direction of the arrows in performing the face massage.

134

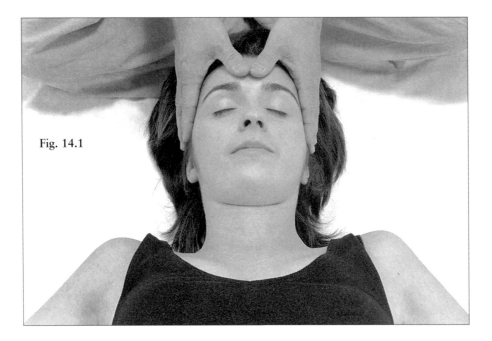

Fig. 14.1

Face Massage

Sit close to the recipient's head. Stroke the side of the recipient's face in a soft and nurturing way. Use your thumbs to massage the forehead from the eyebrows to the hairline (**fig. 14.1**). Use long strokes and move outward toward the side of the face. Finish each stroke by circulating your thumbs on the temples.

Move under the eyes and continue the thumb strokes, smoothing your fingers outward and circulating at the temples. Continue down and below the mouth.

Massage the ears, home to many acupressure points. Rub and squeeze the entire ear, giving special attention to the earlobes. Recipients generally love this! Finish by stroking the side of the recipient's face again.

Adaptation: Applying a drop of aromatherapy oil on your wrists before this movement can feel very nurturing to the recipient. Give a longer facial massage to individuals with a vata constitution.

Precaution: Make sure your hands do not carry the odor of cigarettes, garlic, or any other strong scent. It is not a bad idea to wash your hands just before the facial massage. Some of my students wipe their hands with a mixture of water and tea tree oil on a hand towel that they keep nearby. If you have sweaty hands, use a towel to wipe them dry and apply talcum powder or cornstarch. You can also cleanse your hands on the spot with nonscented baby wipes. Do not use aromatic oil if the recipient is using another vibrational medicine, such as a homeopathic remedy or Bach flower remedies.

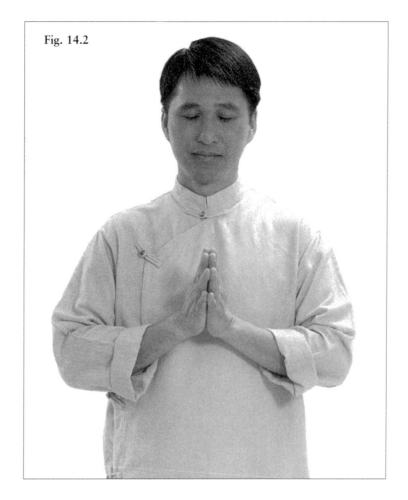

Fig. 14.2

Namaskar

Finish the session as you began, holding your hands in prayer position with a moment of silence. The Namaskar posture develops an attitude of mindfulness and spiritual awareness (**fig. 14.2**). The result is the creation of sacred space. It is an opportunity for the practitioner to be peaceful and cultivate metta, or loving-kindness.

—⁓—

In closing, I would like to say that it has been a great pleasure for me to introduce you to the precious, ancient art of Thai Yoga Massage. As a practitioner of this art, you are part of a rich cultural heritage of Thailand that has lived on through the centuries. The great masters of Thailand who preserved this practice have bestowed a gift of compassionate touch onto the rest of the world. If everyone in the world could practice the art of healing, compassionate touch, we would have peace on earth.

Om mani padme hum! Have a good practice!

APPENDIX 1

Personal Health Questionnaire

Date_____ Time_____

Name_____

Address_____

Phone (home) _____ (work) _____

Age_____ Sex_____ Height_____ Weight_____

Profession_____ Referred by_____

Are you presently taking medications? _____

Which ones? _____

Are you presently under the care of a medical doctor or a health practitioner? _____

If yes, for what reason(s)? _____

Please indicate if you suffer from any of the conditions listed below:

___AIDS

___Allergies

___Aortic aneurysm

___Arteriosclerosis

___Cancer

___Cervical spine problems

___Constipation

___Diarrhea

___Fractures

___Heart disease

___Hemophilia

___Hernia

___High blood pressure

___Joint problems

___Menstruation

___Open wounds and cuts

___Osteoporosis

___Phlebitis (DVT)

___Pregnancy

___Previous dislocation

___Rheumatoid arthritis

___Skin disease

___Stroke

___Surgery

___Other_____

_____

_____

Please circle your problem areas on the drawings above,
and indicate your symptoms with these symbols:

Tension - - - - -   Cramping ////////

Numbness +++++++   Pain >>>>>>>

Do you have any restrictions in movement? _____

Are there any yoga posture(s) or stretch(es) that you fear may be harmful? _____

Are you pregnant? _____ Due date? _____

Do you wear contact lenses? _____ A pacemaker? _____

What physical activities do you regularly participate in? _____

Please detail any recent accidents _____

Please detail any recent surgeries _____

Consent for Thai Yoga Massage

It is understood that the purpose of Thai Yoga Massage is for relaxation and that it is not meant to diagnose or treat any illness, disease, or any other physical or mental disorder, injury, or condition. I have informed my Thai Yoga Massage practitioner about my state of health, and I have transmitted to him/her any recommendations and restrictions on the part of my medical doctor or therapist insofar as Thai Yoga Massage is concerned.

Client's signature_____ Date_____

....

Practitioner's notes

Time spent: _____

Contraindications: _____

Difficulties encountered: _____

Remarks:

Client preferences:

Client dislikes:

APPENDIX 2
Ayurvedic Constitution Questionnaire

*Please circle the appropriate responses. Answers from more than
one row may be applicable.*

	VATA (ACTIVE)	PITTA (PASSIONATE)	KAPHA (SOLID)
Are you usually	Underweight	Medium	Overweight
As a child, were you	Thin	Medium	Plump
Do you have	Light bones and prominent joints	Medium bone structure	Large bone structure
Do you gain weight	With difficulty	Easily, and lose it easily	Easily, and have a hard time losing it
Are your eyes	Small, active, and dark	Of a light color	Large with thick eyelashes
Is your skin	Dry	Freckled	Soft and smooth
Is your complexion	Dark, tans easily	Ruddy, sunburns easily	Fair and pale
Are you	Hyperactive	Active	Slow
Is your digestion	Irregular—sometimes good, sometimes bad	Usually good	Generally slow

Do you	Dislike routine	Can work with routine and a plan	Work well with routine
Are you	A creative thinker	A good initiator and leader	Good at keeping a project running smoothly
Are you sexually	Very active or very inactive	Passionate and domineering	Constant and loyal
Do you like	Travel, art, esoteric subjects	Sports, politics, luxury	Quiet, business, good food
Do you dislike	Cold, wind, and dryness	Heat and midday sun	Cold and dampness
Your memory is	Average	Excellent	Good
Do you speak	Fast	Loud	Melodically
Do you sleep	Lightly	Usually well	Heavily and soundly
When handling money, are you	Wasteful	Methodical	Thrifty
Is your perspiration	Sparse and odorless	Heavy with a strong odor	Heavy with a pleasant odor
Are your bowel movements	Irregular, hard, dry and constipated	Easy and regular; loose stool once to twice a day	Regular, daily, steady, thick and heavy
Is your nose	Small	Medium	Large
Are your fingers	Small, long	Regular	Wide, square shaped
Are your hands/ feet	Cold and dry	Warm and pink	Cool and damp
Do you prefer	Warm climates	Cool and well-ventilated places	Any climate that is not too humid
Are you	Moody, with changeable ideas	Forceful about expressing your ideas	Steady, reliable, slow to change
Is your hair	Rough, wiry, curly	Thin, straight, oily	Thick and wavy
Are your feet	Small, narrow	Medium	Large, wide
Are your facial features	Irregular	Prominent	Round
Are your nails	Brittle	Soft	Strong and thick
Is your chest	Flat	Normally developed	Fully developed
Evaluation	**Vata total:**	**Pitta total:**	**Kapha total:**

Resources

THAI MASSAGE SCHOOLS

There are many schools of Thai massage today, with new ones opening up regularly. However, the quality of teaching varies from school to school. The following resources are ones that I have had direct contact with or that have been highly recommended to me. This is by no means an exhaustive list.

Thailand

The Foundation of Shivago Komarpaj
Old Medical Hospital, near Chiang Mai Cultural Centre
Wualai Road, Chiang Mai, Thailand

This well-established school is the holder of the northern style of Thai massage. The school also runs a healing massage clinic. Classes are given in English, and a twelve-day certificate program is offered.

Thai Traditional Massage School
Wat Po, 2, Sanamchai Rd.
Bangkok, Thailand

This historical massage school has been in operation for the past few centuries. If you can bear with the noisy and crowded temple setting, this school is one of the most respected in Thailand.

North America

Lotus Palm School
Kam Thye Chow
5870 Waverly Street
Montreal, Quebec
Canada H2T 2Y3
Phone: 514.270.5713
www.lotuspalm.com
lotuspalm@hotmail.com

Regular workshops are conducted by the author and qualified teachers internationally. Emphasis is on structural alignment, transitional dance, the implementation of Ayurveda, meditation, and metta practice.

The Center for Thai Yoga Therapy
Saul David Raye
PO Box 903
Topanga, California 90290
Phone: 310.313.5076
www.thaiyoga.com
info@thaiyoga.com

Saul integrates Thai massage with other techniques and practices, including Ayurveda, Hatha yoga, restorative yoga, and pranic healing. Residential training programs and weekend workshops offered.

International Professional School of Bodywork
Pacific College of Oriental Medicine
Richard Gold Ph.D., L.Ac.
San Diego, California
Phone: 800.748.6497 (Int'l School of Bodywork) / 800.729.0491 (Pacific College)
rmgold@znet.com

Dr. Gold teaches northern style Thai Massage (nuad bo'rarn). He has practiced acupuncture and Chinese medicine since 1978.

Europe

The School of Thai Yoga Massage
Kira Balaskas
46A, North View Road
London N8 7LL UK
Phone: 208.3413835
www.thaiyogamassage.co.uk
kira@thaiyogamassage.co.uk

This school regularly runs beginner and advanced diploma trainings in London. The courses are run by Kira Balaskas, an experienced and qualified Thai massage teacher.

MASTER TEACHERS AND PRACTITIONERS

Thailand

Asokananda
The Sunshine Network
149, Kaew Nawarat Soi 4
Chiang Mai 50000, Thailand
www.infothai.com/thaiyogamassage, www.asokananda.com
asokasunshine@hotmail.com

Asokananda is the author of *The Art of Traditional Thai Massage* and the founder of the Sunshine Network, a group of associations promoting spiritual practice that combine Thai massage, yoga, tai chi chuan, and meditation. The network has partners in Thailand, Germany, Austria, New Zealand, Italy, Croatia, England, and India. Facilities differ considerably from place to place.

Massage Master Pichet Boonthumme
3/3 M.5 T.Bahn Vehn A.Hang Dong
Chiang Mai 50230, Thailand
Phone: 66.53.441.704

This Thai massage master is of the highest caliber and is also a well-respected healer in the Thai community. He attracts students from all over the world for advanced studies.

Master Itthidet Manalat ("Poo")
8, Soi 13, Sirimangkalajarn Road, T. Suthep, A. Muang,
Chiang Mai 50200, Thailand
Phone: 66.53.215.267

This master specializes in sen (energy line) therapeutic massage. He teaches basic and advanced therapy courses.

Master Pradit and Cristina Baroni
24 Kaew Nawarat, Soi 4 (near McCormick Hospital)
5000 Chiang Mai, Thailand
Phone: 053.242.310 / 01.884.81.85
www.sunshinehouse.cjb.net
sunshinehouse_cm@hotmail.com

Pradit and Cristina offer a ten-day traditional Thai massage course with introductory classes in Vipassana meditation and yoga.

India

Prabhat Menon
4-B, Maheswar Dharsan S.V. Road
Santacruz (West), Mumbai 400054
Phone: 0091.250.452595
menonprabhat@rediffmail.com

North America

Lissa Guilbault, LMT
LissaGuilbault@hotmail.com

A Thai Yoga Massage teacher from the Lotus Palm School, Lissa has a private practice in Quebec. She has been a close assistant to Kam Thye for a number of years. Lissa teaches group and private sessions in North America and is proficient in English and French.

Chris Holmes
www.thaiyogaworks.com
thaimassage@care2.com

Chris is a Thai Yoga Massage teacher from the Lotus Palm School. He is a skilled communicator and Kripalu yoga teacher. He is available for private sessions and group training in various locations in the United States.

BOOKS AND THAI YOGA MASSAGE ACCESSORIES

Tai Chi Chuan: Mindfulness in Motion
By Kam Thye Chow, with Asokananda

An introductory book to the thirteen basic postures of tai chi chuan, complete with illustrations and photos. The book provides a comprehensive and easy method for learning this art, while returning us back to the heart of tai chi philosophy.

Thai Yoga Massage Sen (Energy) Line Charts

By Kam Thye Chow

These charts offer a front, side, and back view of the ten Sen lines treated in Thai Yoga Massage. The three 12" x 18" color charts include a helpful key for each line.

Lotus Palm Mat

The Lotus Palm mat is suitable for Thai massage, shiatsu, yoga therapy, and other floorwork practices. Each mat set consists of three pieces: a main mat (83" x 39" x 1"), a side mat (16" x 39" x 1"), and a long pillow (10" x 39" x 2"). Each mat is made of a sheet of dense, compressed foam and has a high-quality, durable cotton cover.

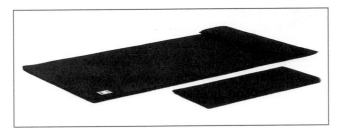

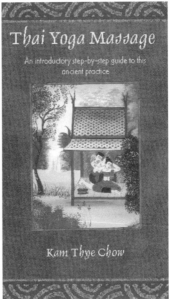

Three strong nylon carrying straps, 2" width with buckle, and a carrying bag (16" x 16" x 40") make the mat easy to transport. Color: burgundy; weight: under 20 pounds.

Thai Yoga Massage video

For those without DVD capacity, Kam Thye Chow offers a step-by-step video that covers the same Thai Yoga Massage techniques in a VHS format. The author guides the viewer through a one-hour full-body massage and demonstrates effective body mechanics and methods for moving with a gentle steady flow.

Thai Yoga Massage CD: Metta

By Uwe Neumann

Featuring original sitar and Sansa music, this beautifully arranged work enhances the rhythmic rocking flow of Thai Yoga Massage.

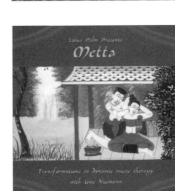

To order books, charts, mat, video, and CD:

www.lotuspalm.com

514.270.5713

Suggested Reading

MASSAGE

Asokananda (Harald Brust). *The Art of Traditional Thai Massage*. Bangkok, Thailand: Editions Duang Kamol, 1994.

——. *Thai Traditional Massage for Advanced Practitioners*. Bangkok, Thailand: Editions Duang Kamol, 1996.

Capellini, Steve, and Michel Van Welden. *Massage for Dummies*. Foster City, Calif.: IDG Books Worldwide, 1999.

Cash, Mel. *Sport and Remedial Massage Therapy*. London: Ebury Press, 1996.

Gold, Richard. *Thai Massage: A Traditional Medical Technique*. Edinburgh: Churchill Livingstone, 1998.

Menon, Prabhat, and Asokananda. *One Rope, Two Feet & Healing Oils: Chavutti Thirummal, The Ancient Art of Keralite Massage*. Bangkok, Thailand: Editions Duang Kamol, 1999.

AYURVEDA

Chopra, Deepak, M.D. *Perfect Health: The Complete Mind/Body Guide*. New York: Harmony Books, 1991.

Frawley, David. *Ayurveda and the Mind: The Healing of Consciousness.* Twin Lakes, Wis.: Lotus Press, 1997.

———. *Yoga & Ayurveda: Self-Healing and Self-Realization.* Twin Lakes, Wis.: Lotus Press, 1999.

Lad, Vasant. *Ayurveda: The Science of Self-Healing. A Practical Guide.* Wilmont, Wis.: Lotus Press, 1985.

Morningstar, Amadea. *Ayurvedic Cooking For Westerners: Familiar Western Food Prepared with Ayurvedic Principles.* Twin Lakes, Wis.: Lotus Press, 1995.

Rhyner, Hans H. *Ayurveda: The Gentle Health System.* New York: Sterling Publishing, 1994.

Warrier, Gopi, and Deepika Gunawant. *The Complete Illustrated Guide to Ayurveda: The Ancient Indian Healing Tradition.* Shaftesbury, Dorset: Element Books, 1997.

YOGA

Asokananda (Harald Brust). *The Yoga of Mindfulness: A Buddhist Path for Body and Mind.* Bangkok, Thailand: Editions Duang Kamol, 1993.

Cope, Stephen. *Yoga and the Quest for the True Self.* New York: Bantam, 1999.

Devi, Nischala Joy. *The Healing Path of Yoga.* New York: Three Rivers Press, 2000.

Desikachar, T. K. V. *The Heart of Yoga: Developing a Personal Practice.* Rochester, Vt.: Inner Traditions International, 1995.

Feuerstein, Georg. *The Yoga Tradition: Its History, Literature, Philosophy and Practice.* Prescott, Ariz.: Hohm Press, 1998.

Myers, Esther. *Yoga & You.* Toronto: Random House, 1996.

Sivananda Yoga Vedanta Center. *Yoga Mind & Body.* London: Dorling Kindersley, 1996.

ANATOMY AND BODY STRUCTURE

Calais-Germain, Blandine. *Anatomy of Movement.* Seattle: Eastland Press, 1993.

———. *Anatomy of Movement: Exercises.* Seattle: Eastland Press, 1996.

Kapit, Wynn, and Lawrence M. Elson. *The Anatomy Coloring Book (2nd ed).* New York: HarperCollins, 1993.

MEDITATION AND PERSONAL GROWTH

Bhikkhu, Buddhadasa. *Mindfulness with Breathing: Unveiling the Secrets of Life.* Chaiya, Thailand: The Dhamma Study and Practice Group, 1989.

Brown, Mick. *The Spiritual Tourist: A Personal Odyssey Through the Outer Reaches of Belief.* New York: Bloomsbury, 1999.

Carlson, Richard. *Don't Sweat the Small Stuff . . . And It's All Small Stuff.* New York: Hyperion, 1997.

Chow, Kam Thye, and Asokananda (Harald Brust). *Tai Chi Chuan: Mindfulness in Motion.* Bangkok, Thailand: Editions Duang Kamol, 1994.

Dalai Lama, H. H., and Howard Cutler. *The Art of Happiness.* New York: Riverhead Books, 1998.

Feldman, Christina, and Jack Kornfield. *Stories of the Spirit, Stories of the Heart.* San Francisco: HarperCollins, 1991.

Khema, Ayya. *I Give You My Life.* Boston and London: Shambhala, 1998.

Rahula, Walpola. *What the Buddha Taught.* New York: Grove Weidenfeld, 1974.

Reid, Daniel. *The Tao of Health, Sex and Longevity: A Modern, Practical Approach to the Ancient Way.* London: Simon & Schuster, 1994.

Snelling, John. *The Buddhist Handbook: A Complete Guide to Buddhist Teaching and Practice.* London: Rider Books, Random House, 1998.

Thich Nhat Hanh. *Old Path White Clouds: Walking in the Footsteps of the Buddha.* Berkeley: Parallax Press, 1991.

———. *Love in Action: Writings on Nonviolent Social Change.* Berkeley: Parallax Press, 1993.

———. *The Heart of the Buddha's Teaching: Transforming Suffering into Peace, Joy and Liberation.* New York: Broadway Books, 1998.

BOOKS OF RELATED INTEREST

The History of Massage
An Illustrated Survey from around the World
by Robert Noah Calvert

Body Rolling
An Experiential Approach to Complete Muscle Release
by Yamuna Zake

The Reflexology Manual
*An Easy-to-Use Illustrated Guide to the Healing Zones
of the Hands and Feet*
by Pauline Wills

Amma Therapy
A Complete Texbook of Oriental Bodywork and Medical Principles
by Tina Sohn and Robert Sohn

Informed Touch
*A Clinician's Guide to the Evaluation and Treatment
of Myofascial Disorders*
by Donna Finando, L.Ac., L.M.T., and Steven Finando, Ph.D., L.Ac.

Soft-Tissue Manipulation
*A Practitioner's Guide to the Diagnosis and Treatment of Soft-Tissue
Dysfunction and Reflex Activity*
by Leon Chaitow, D.O., N.D.

Reiki Energy Medicine
Bringing Healing Touch into Home, Hospital, and Hospice
by Libby Barnett and Maggie Chambers with Susan Davidson

The Handbook of Chinese Massage
Tui Na Techniques to Awaken Body and Mind
by Maria Mercati

Inner Traditions • Bear & Company
P.O. Box 388
Rochester, VT 05767
1-800-246-8648
www.InnerTraditions.com

Or contact your local bookseller